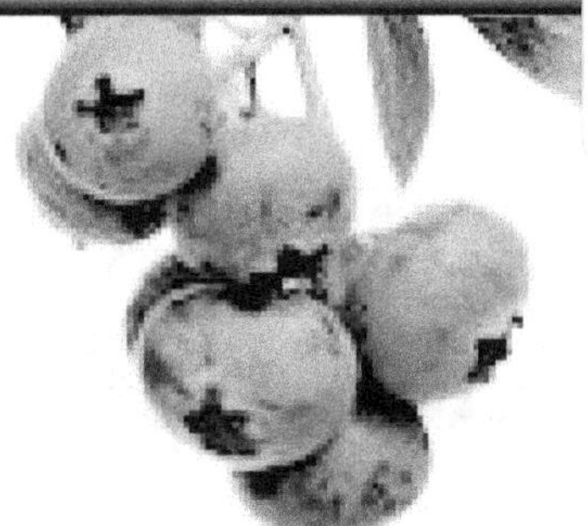

PCOS COOKBOOK

A Culinary
Companion for PCOS
Warriors Offering
50 Recipes, 4 Weeks
Meal Plan for
Hormone Balance,
Fertility Enhancement
& Victory
Celebrations

Allison D. Dixon

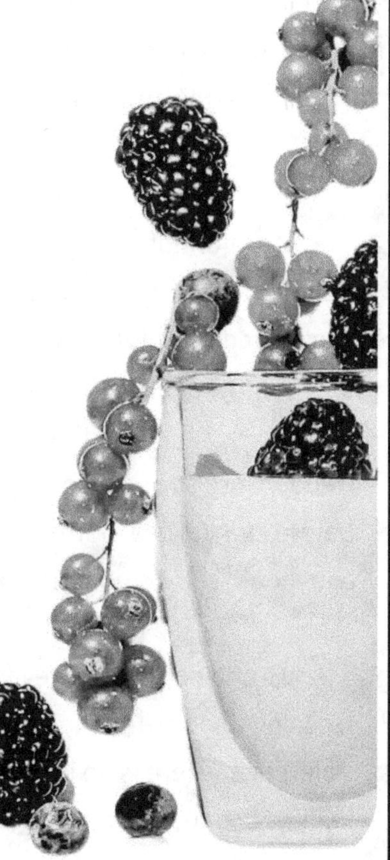

Copyright

©

2024 Allison D. Dixon

Disclaimer:

The information presented in this cookbook is for educational and informational purposes only. While every effort has been made to ensure the accuracy and completeness of the content, the author and publisher assume no responsibility for errors or omissions or for any damages resulting from the use of the information contained herein.

Readers are strongly advised to consult with a qualified health practitioner before making any dietary or lifestyle changes based on the content of this cookbook. The author and publisher disclaim any liability arising directly or indirectly from the use of this cookbook.

Any trademarks, service marks, product names, or named features are assumed to be the property of their respective owners and are used only for reference. There is no implied endorsement if such names are mentioned. Thank you for respecting the intellectual property and legal rights associated with this cookbook.

TABLE OF CONTENTS

TABLE OF CONTENTS

TABLE OF CONTENTS

TABLE OF CONTENTS

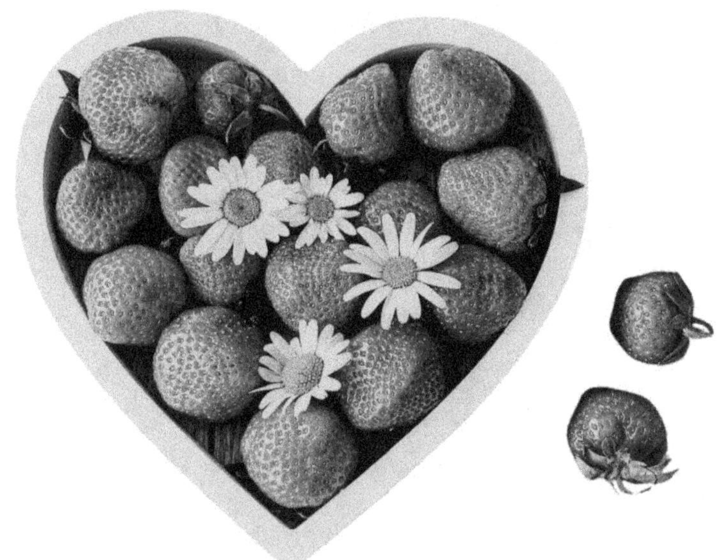

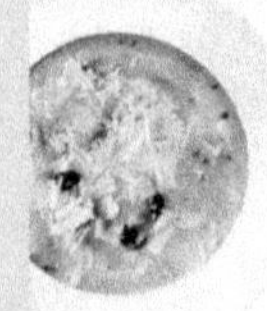 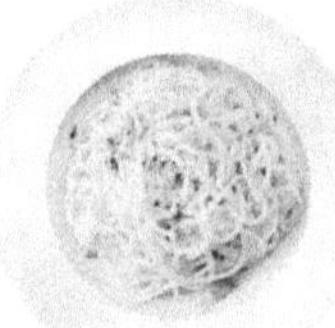 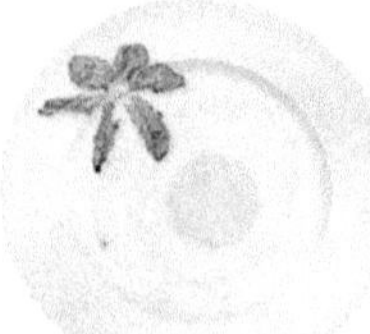 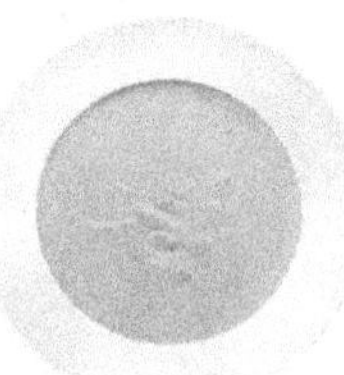 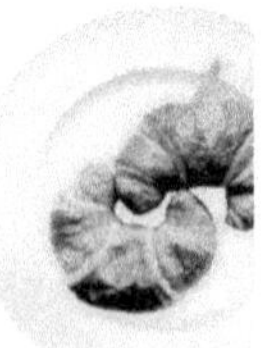

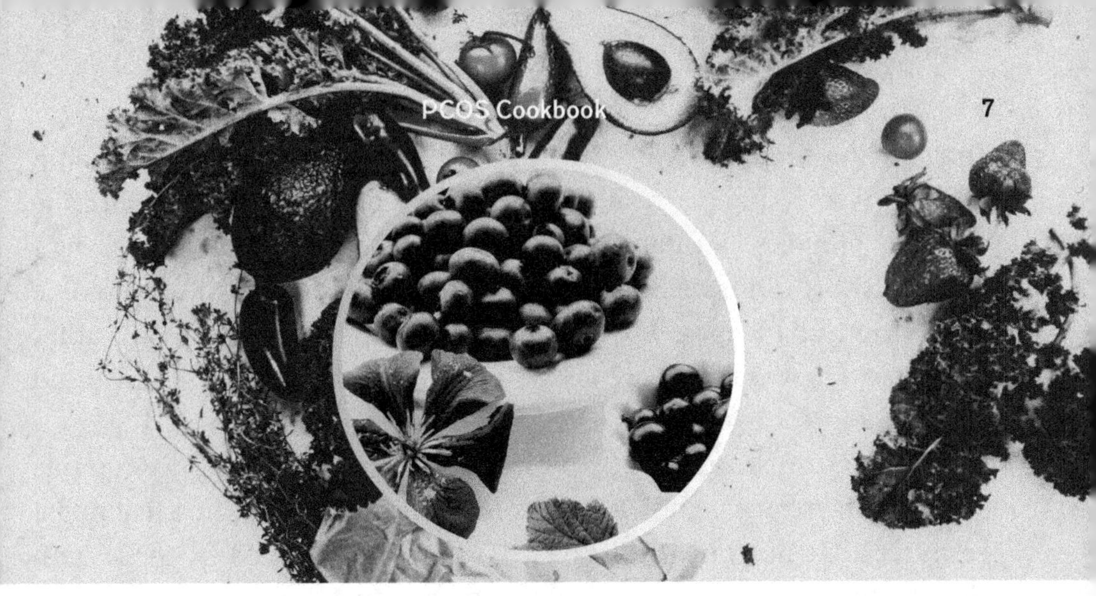

1

INTRODUCTION

1.1: A Personal Journey to PCOS Wellness

AS a dietitian, my professional journey took an unexpected turn when my younger sister, Emma, was diagnosed with Polycystic Ovary Syndrome (PCOS). Witnessing her struggle with the pains and challenges that PCOS brought into her life, I felt compelled to delve into the world of nutrition to understand how a well-crafted diet could become a source of relief and empowerment for those grappling with this condition.

Emma's journey was fraught with frustration, especially when she encountered difficulties in conception. The emotional toll of PCOS manifested in various aspects of her life, prompting me to explore dietary solutions that could potentially alleviate her symptoms and enhance her overall well-being.

Determined to make a difference, I embarked on an extensive research journey, immersing myself in the realms of nutrition and PCOS management. The profound impact of a carefully tailored diet became evident as I discovered how specific food choices could positively influence hormonal balance, weight management, and fertility.

Introducing Emma to a PCOS-friendly diet marked a turning point in her life. Witnessing her resilience and determination, coupled with the positive changes brought about by nutritional adjustments, was nothing short of inspiring. Not only did Emma successfully overcome conception challenges, but she also experienced a myriad of other benefits – increased energy levels, improved mood, and a newfound sense of control over her PCOS symptoms.

It was this transformative experience that motivated me to compile the insights, recipes, and strategies into this cookbook. I envisioned a resource that not only addresses the nutritional needs of those with PCOS but also provides a source of support, understanding, and motivation for anyone navigating the complexities of this condition.

In sharing Emma's story and the wealth of knowledge gathered along the way, my hope is that this cookbook becomes a guide, a companion, and a source of empowerment for individuals facing the challenges of PCOS. Together, let's embark on a journey towards wellness, embracing the transformative power of a nourishing and thoughtful diet.

1.2 Unveiling the World of PCOS

Let's now talk about this health condition that impacts more of us than we realize: Polycystic Ovarian Syndrome (PCOS). I'm not a doctor, but let's go over the essentials.

PCOS in a Nutshell: So, PCOS is like that unexpected visitor at the fertility party, affecting 6% to 12% of reproductive-age women in the U.S. and one in ten in the UK. It's a genuine thing, causing some reproductive issues, but here's the catch: not everyone with PCOS will have fertility problems. Some people may be able to conceive naturally, while others may need medical assistance.

What's the lowdown on PCOS?
Polycystic Ovary Syndrome—that's a mouthful. It disrupts your hormones, causing problems with your menstrual cycle and skin. And, guess what? Many people do not get a diagnosis until they encounter a reproductive issue. It's like playing hide and seek with answers, lasting up to two years and more than three doctor visits.

What causes PCOS and where does it originate? It's a mystery, but it seems that genes, lifestyle, and environment all have a role. High androgen levels are like hormonal rockstars generating all the ruckus, resulting in things like unwanted hair and hair loss.

Then there's the insulin party; some of us develop resistance. Insulin is the blood sugar traffic policeman, but when it is disregarded, disaster strikes. It affects the ovaries, weight, and may even lead to the dreaded type 2 diabetes. As if that wasn't enough, genes play a role, and your family history might influence your PCOS journey.

PCOS may run in families, making it a genetically predisposed condition. Mitochondria, our cells' powerhouses, may also play a role —science is still finding that out. And, hey, your ethnicity could be a factor; some studies suggest that certain ethnic groups are more likely to develop PCOS, each with their own set of symptoms.

That's PCOS in a nutshell! But, hey, always ask the professionals for the genuine deal. This cookbook isn't a miracle panacea, but it does include some yummy dishes and information to help you manage the PCOS rollercoaster. Stay amazing, buddies!

Decoding PCOS: A Real Talk About Symptoms, Diagnosis, and Lifestyle
Okay, let's be serious about PCOS (Polycystic Ovary Syndrome). It's like a tricky puzzle that affects up to 12% of reproductive-age women in the United States, causing some reproductive chaos. Now, I'm not an expert, but let's break down what's going on.

Symptoms Unveiled:
So, PCOS is a bit of a shape-shifter, with symptoms that differ from person to person. Irregular periods? Yeah, it is a classic. Your body can opt to ovulate less often or simply skip the entire process. That entails times of hide and seek, either too often or not at all. And, hey, some report higher-than-normal flows.

Tip: Keep an eye on your cycles, and if anything seems unusual for three months in a row, consult with a professional. They may suggest hormone and fertility testing.

Now, let's speak about skin and hair. Excessive hair growth in unwanted areas, hair loss in desired areas, and a special visitor known as acne. Blame it on the androgens (the testosterone squad) having a party in your body. Oh, and weight gain, particularly in the stomach? PCOS tends to disrupt your metabolism.

Fertility Hurdles: Trying to conceive? PCOS may throw a curveball. Hormonal hiccups may interfere with ovulation, making the process similar to catching a shooting star. And here's the thing: getting diagnosed with PCOS does not signify the end of baby hopes. Many people are still able to conceive without the use of fertility drugs.

PCOS may also lead to mental health problems. Sadness, anxiety – it's like an unwelcome tag-along since coping with symptoms isn't always a stroll in the park.

Diagnosis Details:
No blood test indicates "You have PCOS!" It's more like a detective game for physicians. Your history, symptoms, and a few tests, such as a pelvic ultrasound, may all be on the schedule. It's all about weeding out the impostors.

Fertility and beyond:
Concerned about fertility? PCOS may be difficult to manage, but it does not rule out being a parent. Fertility medicines may be a possibility, but there's good news: studies show that PCOS patients have as many pregnancies and children as those without PCOS.

The Long-Term Health Hustle:

Now, strap on for the long-term health trip. PCOS may cause insulin resistance, type 2 diabetes, obesity, cholesterol issues, and other complications. It's not all doom and gloom, however; a little lifestyle control may go a long way.

Managing PCOS:

There is no treatment for PCOS, but the key is to manage symptoms and health issues. It is a collaborative endeavor comprising hormone specialists, gynecologists, dieticians, and others. Lifestyle changes are essential, such as maintaining a healthy weight and adopting a Mediterranean diet. Consider flexibility and sustainability rather than harsh standards.

So, there you have it: PCOS unpacked. This is a journey, not a sprint. If you have PCOS, remember that you are not alone, and seeking professional advice is always a good idea. Stay amazing, buddies!

1.3 Embracing a PCOS-Friendly Lifestyle: Diet and Exercise Tips

Now, let's discuss the power combination of nutrition and exercise in your PCOS journey. It's not about following precise rules; it's about living a life that makes you happy and works for you.

Step 1: Maintain a Healthy Weight. It's like encouraging your body to have regular cycles and ovulate on its own. Talk with your doctor about your optimal weight. They may use words like BMI (Body Mass Index), but keep in mind that there is no one-size-fits-all approach. Your level of activity and ethnicity are other important considerations.

Experts advise losing 5-10% of your body weight will help alleviate discomfort and increase your chances of conceiving.

Step 2: Eat Smarter and Move More:

Now, here's the deal: reducing weight with PCOS isn't always easy. Crash diets? Nah, they may do more damage than benefit. What you need is a comprehensive strategy, including a healthy diet and frequent exercise. It's not about deprivation; it's about making decisions that benefit you.

Step 3: What is on the PCOS Menu?:

So, let's discuss the PCOS diet. Consider tailoring, flexibility, and sustainability. Say welcome to Mediterranean-style delights, including whole grains, fiber-rich sweets, healthy fats, and protein-packed marvels. Replace high-GI carbohydrates with low-GI carbs, and reduce your consumption of sugary processed foods. Balance is the name of the game.

Step 4: Exercise: Find Your Groove:

Regarding exercise, there is no one-size-fits-all golden recipe. It's not about following what everyone else is doing; it's about discovering what works for you. Whether it's running, walking, cycling, or swimming, choose something you like. If weight reduction is your objective, include some resistance activities. Yoga and pilates? They are more than simply stretching exercises; they are also stress relievers.

The bottom line:

It's not a sprint, but a marathon. PCOS is a journey, and food and exercise are your constant companions. Your decisions are important, so be gentle to yourself. Adopt a healthy lifestyle that benefits both your body and spirit. And, hey, always include the professionals; they've got your back on this expedition.

1.4 Unlocking PCOS Wellness: A Recipe for a Vibrant Life

Hey, PCOS fighters! Before you embark on your cookbook excursion, be assured that the dishes are more than simply tasty; they were created with your PCOS journey in mind.

Why recipes in this cookbook shine:
Every meal is a combination of tastes and nutrients that are compatible with PCOS control. Consider this: whole grains for consistent energy, high-fiber marvels to keep things going smoothly, healthy fats as the star, and protein-rich goodies to power your day.

Meeting PCOS requirements:
What's on your plate is important, and our recipes do it right. They tick every PCOS box:

1. **Balanced Goodness**: Tailored to your dietary preferences, with an emphasis on sustainability.

2. **Mediterranean Magic**: Inspired by the rich, PCOS-friendly Mediterranean diet, which includes whole grains, high fiber, healthy fats, and high-quality protein sources.

3. **Low GI Swaps**: We've got you covered with swaps that substitute high-glycemic-index (GI) carbohydrates with low-GI alternatives.

4. **Sweets the Smart Way**: We understand the sugary temptations, which is why our recipes limit the sweetness and avoid manufactured sugary traps.

5. **Blood Sugar Buddy**: We've intelligently mixed proteins and carbohydrates to keep blood sugar levels stable and help you manage PCOS symptoms.

Why Trust Our Recipes?
Your health journey is important, and we have your back. The recipes in this collection are more than simply meals; they are about creating a lifestyle that is compatible with PCOS treatment.

So, put on your apron and prepare to relish every mouthful, knowing that these recipes will make your PCOS journey a little sweeter and a lot healthier. Happy cooking!

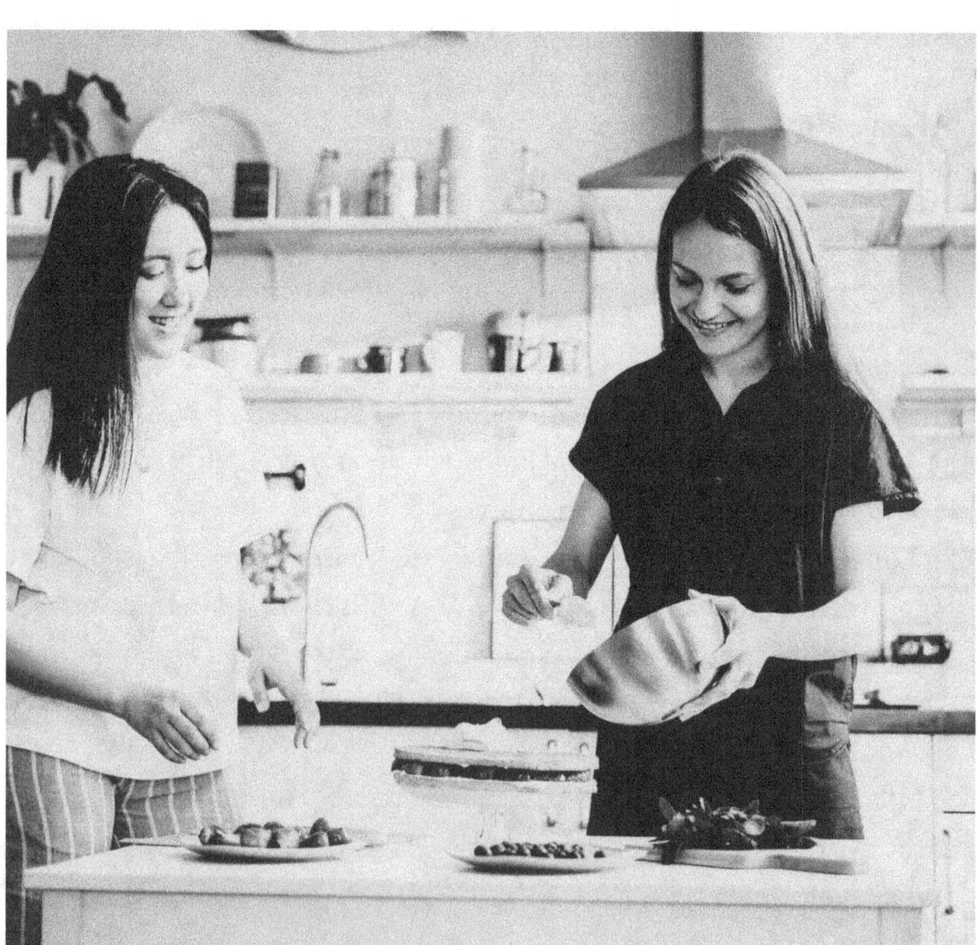

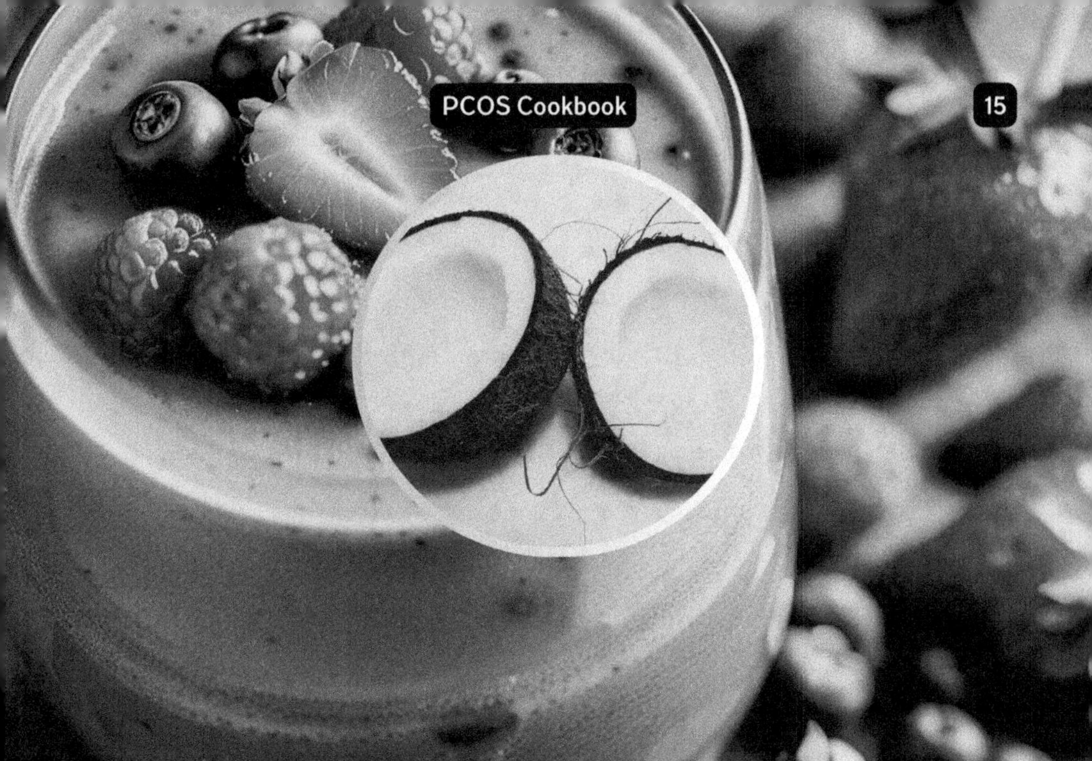

Tasty PCOS management smoothie

2

BREAKFAST DELIGHTS

Good morning champs! ☀ Welcome to the breakfast extravaganza, where we'll delve into a quintet of morning enchantment. I'll be your guide on this flavor-packed excursion, and I guarantee it will be a wonderful ride. Get ready for Berry Smoothie Bowl, Avocado and Egg Toast, the delectable Greek Yogurt Parfait, Quinoa morning Bowl, and the show-stopping Veggie Omelette Delight.

We're going to start the day with a breakfast fiesta that's both delicious and nutritious. Let's get the blenders going, toasters toasting, quinoa cooking, and eggs sizzling - breakfast is ready! 🍓🥑🥄

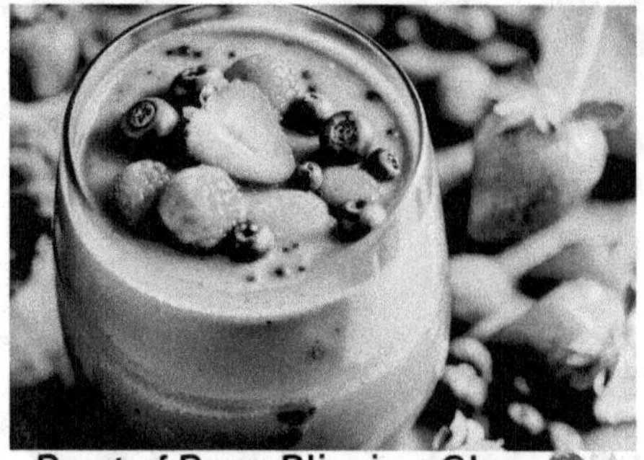

Burst of Berry Bliss in a Glass 🍓✨

Prep ⏰	**Cook** ⏰	**Serves**
5 minutes	Raw	1

Smoothie with Triple Berries

This is my favorite smoothie, and it's ideal for treating PCOS.
Berries are among the lowest GI fruits, so feel free to include them into your smoothie. You even get your daily dosage of greens. It makes an excellent quick breakfast on the road or a healthful afternoon snack.

INGREDIENTS:

- Two cups of liquid (water, almond milk, etc.).
- ½ frozen banana
- 2 cup frozen organic berries (blackberries, raspberries, and blueberries)
- 1 tablespoon chia seeds.
- A handful of spinach.
- coconut shavings (optional)
- Walnuts are optional.
- If you want it cold, add a few ice cubes!

INSTRUCTIONS

1. Simply put all ingredients in a blender.
2. Pour into a large glass.
3. Sprinkle with coconut and walnuts (optional).
4. Enjoy!

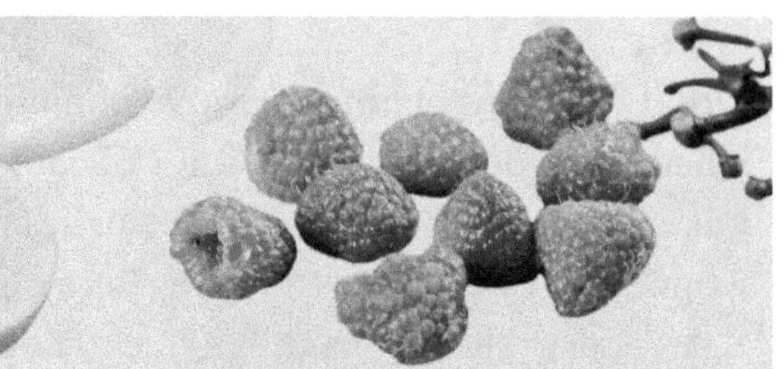

Strawberries

This refreshing Triple Berry Smoothie is not only delicious, but it's also PCOS-friendly. It's your go-to quick breakfast or healthy afternoon pick-me-up, packed with berry sweetness and a hint of greens. With a mix of frozen banana, organic berries, chia seeds, spinach, and optional coconut shavings or walnuts, it's a delectable treat that won't keep you confined to the kitchen. Simply combine all of the ingredients in a blender, give it a spin, and you'll have a tasty PCOS management drink! 🍓🥛

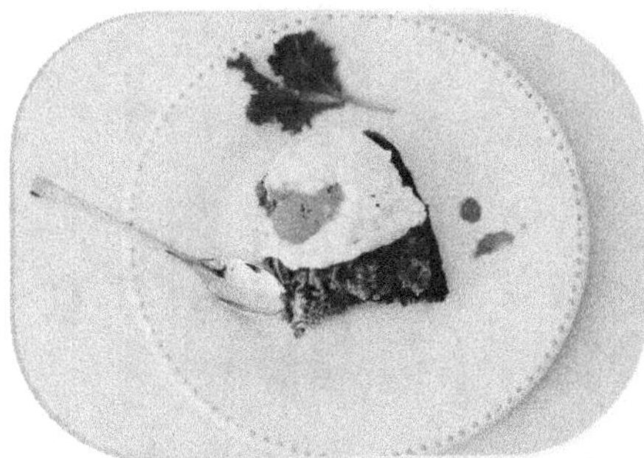

Avocado + Egg Toast Magic! 🥑🔍

Avocado and Egg Toast: A Breakfast Delight

Morning Vibes:

Hello, fellow breakfast-lovers! Let's talk about the avocado and egg toast, which is a breakfast game-changer. It's more than just your typical breakfast; it's a flavor and nutrient explosion that will make your day.

INGREDIENTS:

- One slice of whole-grain bread
- 1 ripe avocado
- 1 egg
- Salt and pepper to taste
- Optional toppings: red pepper flakes, feta cheese, or a dash of hot sauce

INSTRUCTIONS

1. Toast the whole-grain bread until it tastes good.
2. Mash the ripe avocado and spoon it equally over the toasted slice of bread while it's toasting.
3. Cook the egg in a different pan to your desired doneness, either sunny-side up or over easy.
4. Gently slide the fried egg onto the toast that has been topped with avocado.
5. Add salt and pepper for seasoning, along with any extra toppings you choose.
6. Savor the ideal balance of flavors by diving in while it's still warm.

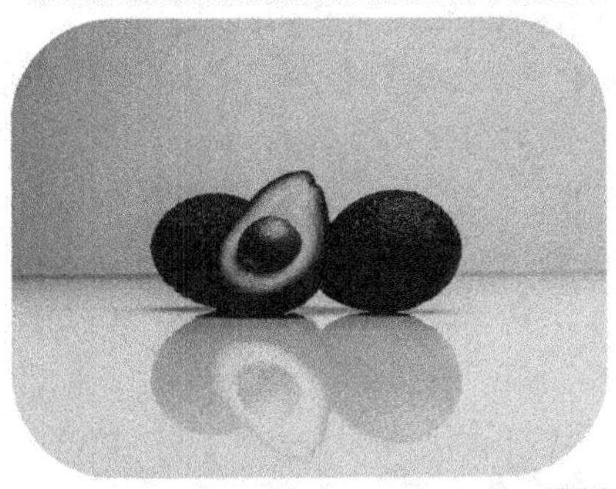

Avocado love in a snapshot. 🥑🤍

So let's toast to mornings improved by avocado and egg. It's too amazing to skip for breakfast—creamy, flavorful, and PCOS-friendly. One mouthwatering meal at a time, be ready to tackle your day! 🥑🔍

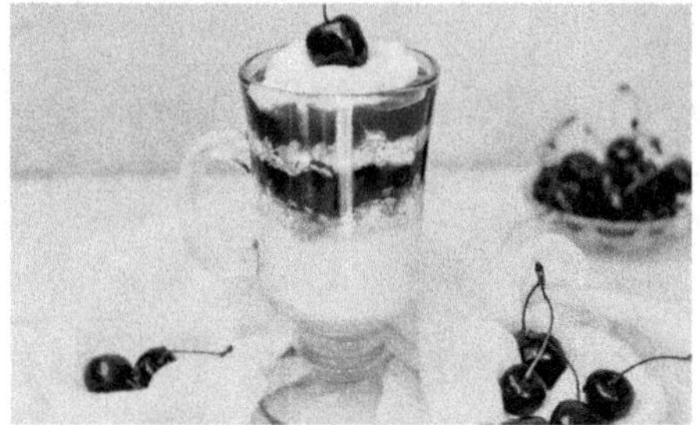

Parfait perfection.

Greek Yogurt Parfait: My Morning Glory

Prep ⏰ 10 minutes   **Cook** ⏰ 0 Minutes   **Serves** 1

Hi there, lovers of breakfast! Here's a treat that's perfect for anyone with PCOS: my very own Greek Yogurt Parfait. It's a celebration of tastes and nutrients that will give you the best start to the day—it's more than simply a parfait.

This parfait is about providing your body with the nutrition it needs, not only about taste.

INGREDIENTS:

- 1 cup of dairy-free yogurt or unsweetened Greek yogurt
- 1/4 cup of finely chopped almonds or walnuts
- 1/4 cup of raw blueberries
- 1/4 cup of raspberries, fresh
- 1/4 cup sliced fresh strawberries
- 1 tablespoon ground flaxseed
- 1 tablespoon unsweetened shredded coconut
- 1 teaspoon honey or other natural sweetener (optional)

That's my veggie omelette delight that is suitable for those with PCOS. A morning wonder that will satisfy your palate and support your wellness goals. It's a protein-rich, vegetable-rich breakfast that's easy to make and sets the stage for a great day. Savor your vegetable-filled bliss!

INSTRUCTIONS

1. To start, fill a glass or jar with a thick layer of unsweetened Greek yogurt or your favorite dairy-free substitute at the bottom to form a strong protein base.
2. Next, add a layer of chopped almonds or walnuts to your parfait for a wonderful crunch and to add healthy fats.
3. Next, let's add a layer of fresh blueberries and raspberries to add some color and antioxidants, making a colorful and nutrient-rich stratum.
4. Add another dollop of yogurt—who could resist having more of that deliciously creamy substance?
5. Add the shredded coconut, crushed flaxseed, and strawberries in slices to create a trio of nutrient-dense treats.
6. Continue making these delectable layers until you've used every wonderful item. Finish by adding a final layer of yogurt on top.
7. Sprinkle a teaspoon of honey or another natural sweetener on top if you're feeling particularly sugary.

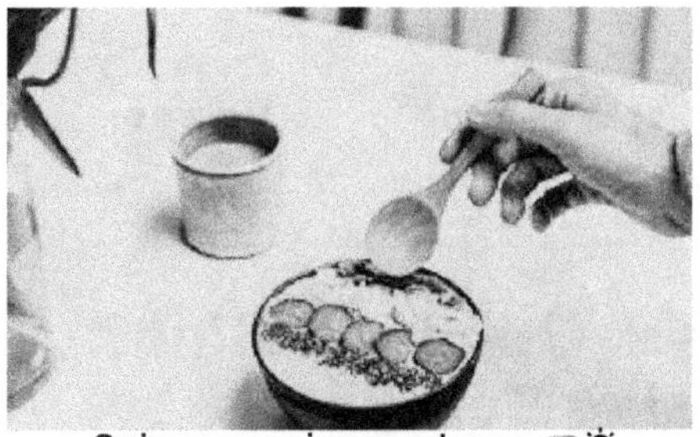

Quinoa morning goodness. 🥣☀️

Prep ⏰	Cook ⏰	Serves
5 minutes	20 Minutes	1

Quinoa Breakfast Bowl: A Morning Marvel

Greetings, lovers of breakfast! Prepare yourself for my PCOS Quinoa Breakfast Bowl, the next great morning marvel. It's a nutritional powerhouse designed to up your breakfast game, not just a bowl.

INGREDIENTS:

- 1/2 cup quinoa
- 1 cup unsweetened almond milk or your preferred dairy-free alternative
- 1/4 cup sliced almonds
- 1/4 cup fresh strawberries, diced
- 1/4 cup banana slices
- 1 tablespoon chia seeds
- 1 tablespoon pure maple syrup or a natural sweetener (optional)
- A pinch of cinnamon for that extra warmth

Here it is: my Quinoa Breakfast Bowl. A delicious breakfast treat that complements your wellness path while also tempting your taste senses. Easy to prepare, full of healthy deliciousness, and sure to make your mornings wonderful. Savor the nutrient-rich adventure that lies ahead! 🥣🍓

INSTRUCTIONS

1. Rinse the quinoa thoroughly under cold water.
2. In a saucepan, combine the rinsed quinoa and unsweetened almond milk. Bring it to a boil, then reduce the heat, cover, and simmer for 15-20 minutes or until the quinoa is cooked and has absorbed the liquid.
3. While the quinoa is simmering, toast the sliced almonds in a dry skillet over medium heat until golden brown and fragrant. Keep an eye on them to prevent burning.
4. Once the quinoa is cooked, fluff it with a fork and transfer it to a bowl.
5. Top the quinoa with sliced almonds, fresh strawberries, banana slices, and chia seeds.
6. Drizzle with pure maple syrup or your preferred natural sweetener if you desire a touch of sweetness.
7. Sprinkle a pinch of cinnamon for that cozy flavor.

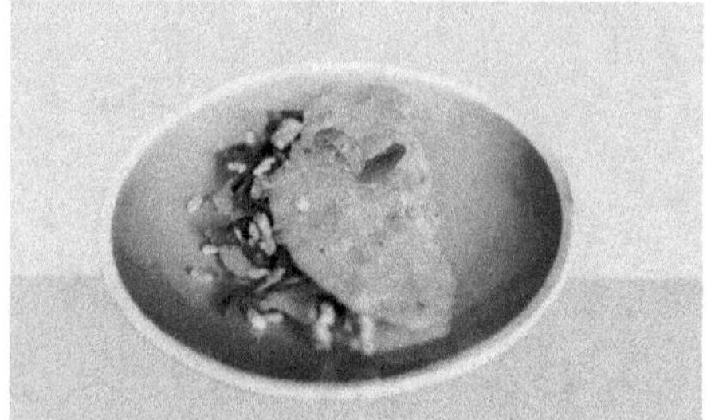

Veggie omelet delight.

Veggie Omelet Delight: Morning Sunshine

Prep ⏰	Cook ⏰	Serves
10 minutes	5 Minutes	1

Good morning, breakfast champions! Prepare for my PCOS-friendly Veggie Omelet Delight, a morning sensation. It's a symphony of vegetables and protein, expertly prepared to start your day with a taste and nutrition boost. It's more than just an omelet.

INGREDIENTS:

- 2 large eggs
- 1/4 cup bell peppers, diced (mix of colors for a vibrant plate)
- 1/4 cup spinach, chopped
- 1/4 cup tomatoes, diced
- 1/4 cup mushrooms, sliced
- 1/4 cup feta cheese, crumbled
- 1 tablespoon olive oil
- Salt and pepper to taste
- Fresh herbs (like chives or parsley) for garnish

Here it is: my Quinoa Breakfast Bowl. A delicious breakfast treat that complements your wellness path while also tempting your taste senses. Easy to prepare, full of healthy deliciousness, and sure to make your mornings wonderful. Savor the nutrient-rich adventure that lies ahead! 🥣🍓

INSTRUCTIONS

1. In a bowl, whisk the eggs until well beaten. Season with a pinch of salt and pepper.
2. Heat olive oil in a non-stick skillet over medium heat.
3. Add diced bell peppers, chopped spinach, diced tomatoes, and sliced mushrooms to the skillet. Sauté until the veggies are tender.
4. Pour the beaten eggs over the sautéed veggies, ensuring an even distribution.
5. Allow the omelet to set at the edges. As it starts to firm up, gently lift the edges with a spatula to let the uncooked eggs flow underneath.
6. Once the eggs are mostly set, sprinkle crumbled feta cheese over one half of the omelet.
7. Fold the other half over the cheesy delight, creating a semi-circle omelet.
8. Cook for an additional minute until the cheese melts, and the omelet is cooked to perfection.
9. Slide onto a plate, garnish with fresh herbs, and serve hot.

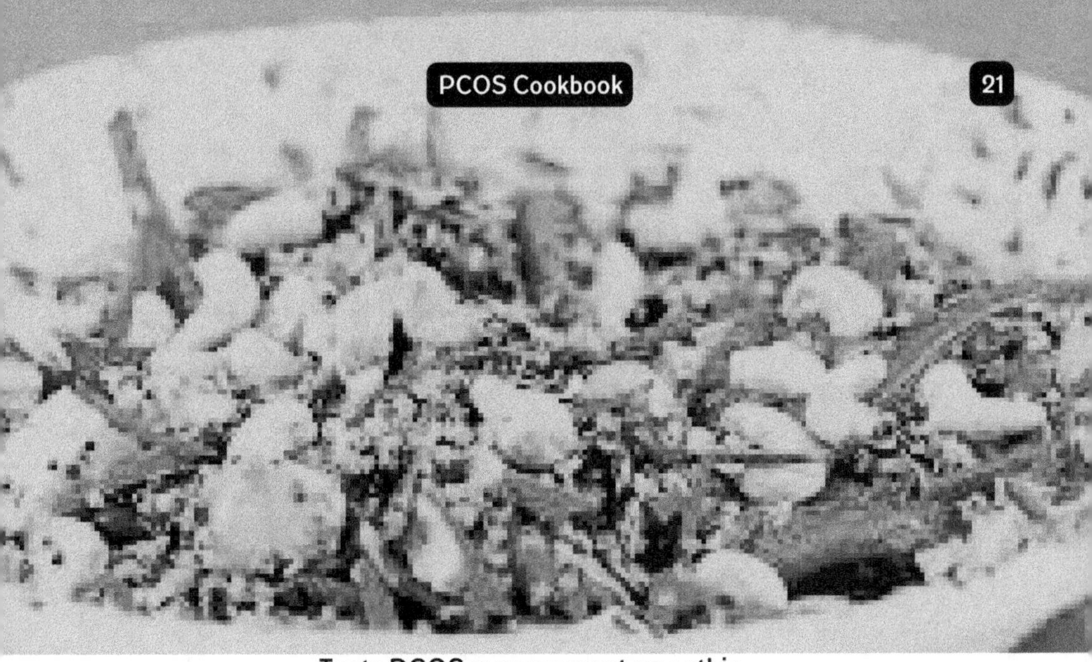

Tasty PCOS management smoothie

3

ENERGIZING STARTERS

MY Kickstart to Vibrant Mornings!

Hey, breakfast enthusiasts! Welcome to the Energizing Starters section – my secret weapon for vibrant mornings. These recipes are not just starters; they're power-packed creations designed to kickstart your day with energy and flavor.

Get ready to indulge in a delightful PCOS-friendly quartet: Quinoa Salad with Roasted Veggies, Spinach and Feta Stuffed Mushrooms, Sweet Potato and Chickpea Patties, Berry Nutty Overnight Oats, and Tomato Avocado Bruschetta. Let's embark on a flavorful journey that not only satisfies your taste buds but also nourishes your body with the goodness it deserves. Let's energize those mornings! 🍽🍴

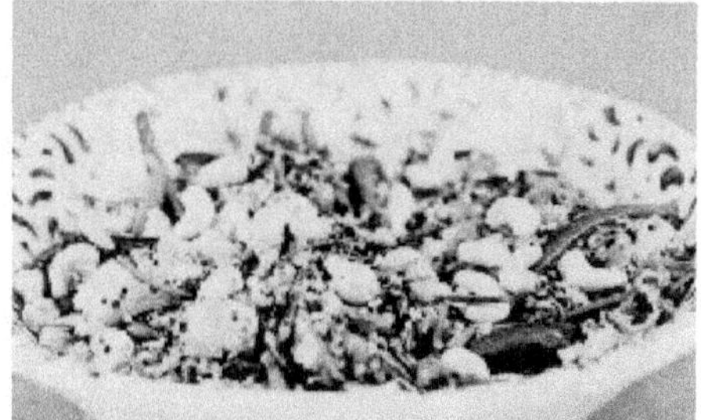

Quinoa Veggie Delight.

Prep ⏰	Cook ⏰	Serves
15 minutes	20 Minutes	2

Quinoa Salad with Roasted Veggies

Hello, lovers of breakfast! Have you ever yearned for a breakfast that not only tantalizes your taste senses but also provides you with goodness to fuel your day—especially if you have PCOS? You don't need to search any farther since my PCOS-friendly Quinoa Salad with Roasted Veggies will revolutionize your morning routine. It's a colorful beginning to a colorful day, not just a salad!

INGREDIENTS:

- 1 cup quinoa
- 2 cups mixed veggies (bell peppers, cherry tomatoes, zucchini – let your creativity run wild!)
- 2 tablespoons olive oil
- 1 teaspoon dried herbs (rosemary, thyme, or your favorites)
- Salt and pepper to taste
- 1/4 cup feta cheese (optional; choose a PCOS-friendly cheese or skip if lactose-sensitive)
- Fresh herbs for garnish (optional)

INSTRUCTIONS

1. Rinse the quinoa under cold water. Cook it according to package instructions, and let it cool.
2. Preheat your oven to a toasty 400°F (200°C). While it's warming up, chop your veggies into bite-sized pieces.
3. Toss the veggies with olive oil, dried herbs, salt, and pepper. Spread them on a baking sheet and let them roast in the oven until they're beautifully golden and tender.
4. Once your quinoa and veggies are ready, combine them in a bowl. Add that PCOS-friendly cheese or skip for a dairy-free option.
5. Give it a good toss to marry the flavors, and garnish with fresh herbs if you're feeling fancy.

Here it is: my Quinoa Salad with Roasted Vegetables, suitable for those with PCOS. A breakfast meal that has the appearance and flavor of a masterpiece. It's the colorful jumpstart you deserve, loaded with flavor, nutrition, and goodness that's ideal for PCOS. Chew on this bowl of blissful morning food! Happy PCOS-Friendly Breakfast

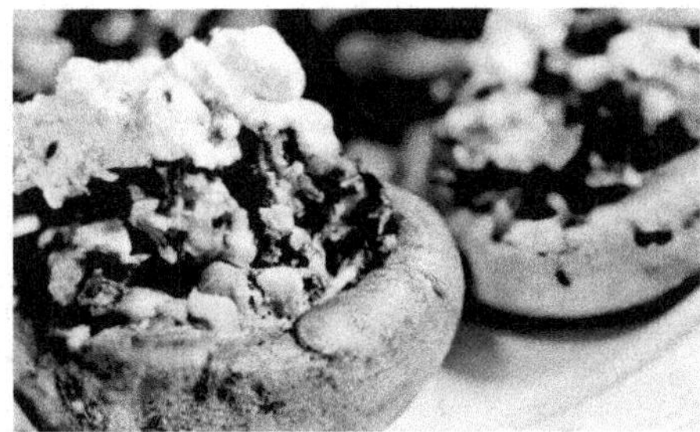

Spinach Feta Mushrooms delight! 🍄

Prep ⏱	Cook ⏱	Serves
15 minutes	20 Minutes	2

Spinach and Feta Stuffed Mushrooms

Hi there, lovers of breakfast! My next recipe for a tasty and PCOS-friendly breakfast delight is Spinach and Feta Stuffed Mushrooms. Imagine this: savory mushrooms that are stuffed with a delicious combination of spinach and feta, brightening your morning and satisfying your palate.

INGREDIENTS:

- 6 large mushrooms, stems removed
- 1 cup fresh spinach, finely chopped
- 1/2 cup feta cheese (choose a PCOS-friendly cheese or skip if lactose-sensitive)
- 1 clove garlic, minced
- 1 tablespoon olive oil
- Salt and pepper to taste
- Fresh herbs for garnish (because we eat with our eyes too)

Here it is: my PCOS-friendly stuffed mushrooms with spinach and feta. A delicious treat that fits your PCOS-friendly lifestyle while also satisfying your palate. Get your day started with a delicious and wholesome taste. Cheers to happy, joyful mornings! Happy PCOS-Friendly Mornings! 🍄⚙️

INSTRUCTIONS

1. Preheat your oven to a cozy 375°F (190°C). It's about to get aromatic in your kitchen!
2. In a pan, sauté the chopped spinach and minced garlic with a splash of olive oil until the spinach wilts. Season with a pinch of salt and pepper.
3. While your spinach mix is cooling, lightly brush the mushroom caps with olive oil and place them on a baking sheet.
4. In a bowl, combine the sautéed spinach mix with feta cheese. This is your flavorful stuffing!
5. Generously stuff each mushroom cap with the spinach and feta mix. It's like creating little beds of joy.
6. Pop those stuffed mushrooms into the preheated oven for around 15-20 minutes or until they're golden brown and oozing with deliciousness.

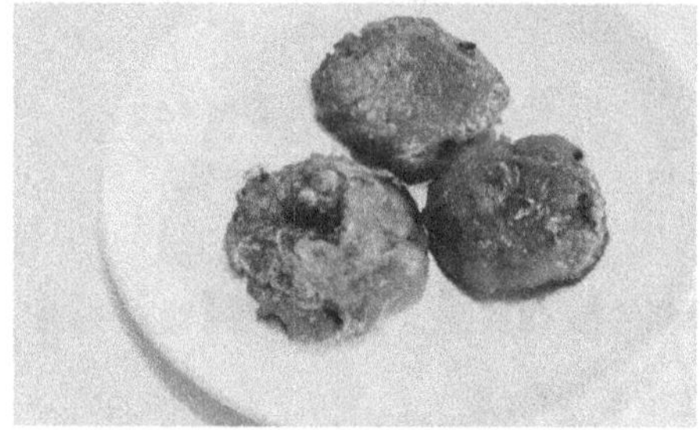

Sweet Potato Chickpea Patties. 🍠

Prep ⏰	Cook ⏰	Serves
15 minutes	15 Minutes	2

Sweet Potato and Chickpea Patties

Hi! Here is another delicious delicacy that is suitable for people with PCOS: my sweet potato and chickpea patties. Picture golden-brown patties that are oozing with sweet potato and chickpea deliciousness. A lovely way to start your morning, it has a combination of flavors and ingredients that are good for PCOS.

INGREDIENTS:

- 1 large sweet potato, peeled and grated
- 1 can (15 oz) chickpeas, drained and mashed
- 1/2 cup rolled oats (choose gluten-free oats for a PCOS-friendly option)
- 1/4 cup finely chopped red onion
- 1 teaspoon ground cumin
- 1 teaspoon paprika
- Salt and pepper to taste
- Olive oil for cooking
- Greek yogurt or a PCOS-friendly alternative for serving

INSTRUCTIONS

1. Preheat your skillet or pan over medium heat. We're getting ready to sizzle!
2. In a large bowl, combine grated sweet potato, mashed chickpeas, rolled oats, chopped red onion, ground cumin, paprika, salt, and pepper. Mix until everything plays well together.
3. Shape the mixture into patties. The size is up to you – go for your preferred patty perfection.
4. Drizzle some olive oil in your preheated pan and cook those patties until they're golden and crispy on each side. It's like creating flavor-packed sunshine on a plate.
5. Serve these beauties with a dollop of Greek yogurt or your favorite PCOS-friendly alternative. Get ready for a taste explosion!

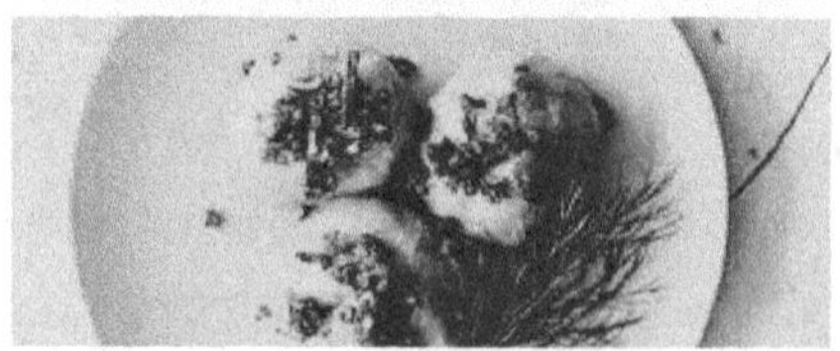

Here you have it - my sweet potato and chickpea patties that are suitable for people with PCOS. A breakfast feast that fits your PCOS-friendly quest while also satisfying your palate. Savor the flavors of a PCOS-friendly morning and indulge in the crispy, golden bliss! 🍠 #PCOSFriendlyFeastt

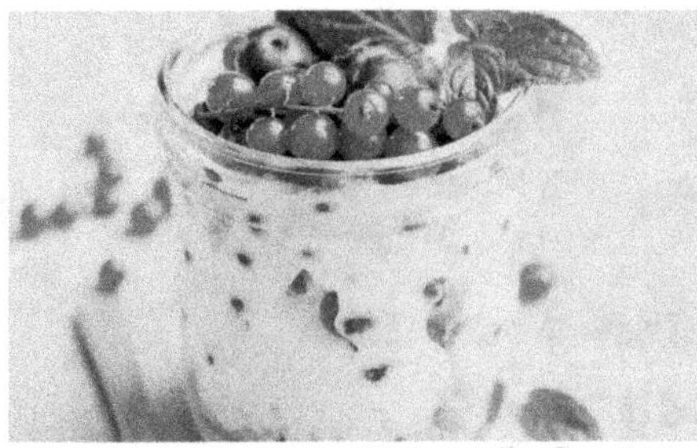

A breakfast dream. 🍓🥜

Prep ⏰	Cook ⏰	Serves
5 minutes	0 Minutes	1

Berry Nutty Overnight Oats

Hey breakfast enthusiasts! Prepare to transform your mornings with my Berry Nutty Overnight Oats, a PCOS-friendly treat. This dish is more than simply a bowl of oatmeal; it's an ode to berries, almonds, and everything wonderful that helps you on your path to PCOS wellness. Come on, let's tuck into some morning bliss!

INGREDIENTS:

- 1/2 cup rolled oats (choose gluten-free oats for a PCOS-friendly option)
- 1/2 cup unsweetened almond milk or any PCOS-friendly milk alternative
- 1/4 cup Greek yogurt or a PCOS-friendly alternative
- 1/2 cup mixed berries (blueberries, raspberries, strawberries – pick your favorites!)
- 1 tablespoon chia seeds
- 1 tablespoon chopped nuts (walnuts, almonds – go nuts!)
- 1 teaspoon honey or a natural sweetener (optional, depending on your sweetness preference)
- A pinch of cinnamon for extra flavor (optional)

INSTRUCTIONS

1. In a jar or container, combine rolled oats, almond milk, Greek yogurt, chia seeds, and a drizzle of honey if you're in the mood for sweetness. Mix it up!
2. Add your chosen mix of berries and give it another good stir. This is where the magic starts to happen.
3. Seal the jar or cover the container and let it chill in the refrigerator overnight. It's like a cozy slumber party for your oats and berries.
4. The next morning, give your oats a gentle mix. Top it with chopped nuts for that delightful crunch.
5. If you're feeling adventurous, sprinkle a pinch of cinnamon for an extra burst of flavor.

There you have it – Berry Nutty Overnight Oats. A wonderful morning routine that fits your PCOS-friendly lifestyle while also satisfying your palate. Enjoy a bowl of goodies to get your day off to a berry-licious start! 🍓🥥

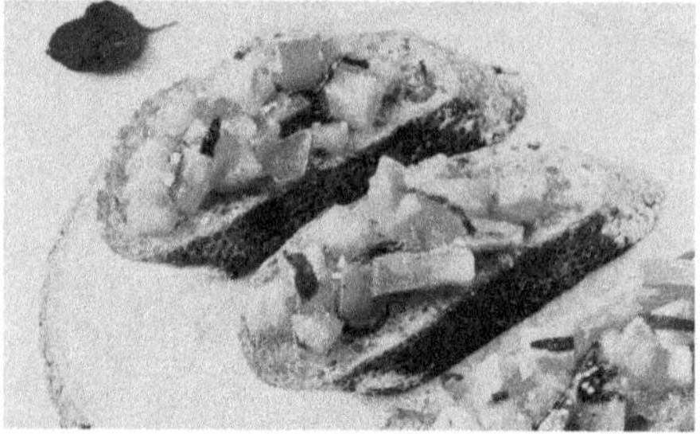

Tomato Avocado Bruschetta perfection.

Prep ⏰	Cook ⏰	Serves
10 minutes	5 Minutes	2

Tomato Avocado Bruschetta

Hello, foodies! The PCOS-friendly Tomato Avocado Bruschetta is the grand conclusion of our Energizing Starters, so get ready. It's more than just a snack—it's a flavor explosion with a PCOS-friendly twist. Prepare to experience a new level of flavor!

INGREDIENTS:

- 1 cup cherry tomatoes, diced
- 1 ripe avocado, diced
- 1 clove garlic, minced
- 2 tablespoons fresh basil, chopped
- 1 tablespoon extra virgin olive oil
- 1 teaspoon balsamic vinegar (optional)
- Salt and pepper to taste
- Slices of whole-grain or gluten-free bread (choose a PCOS-friendly option)

This is it: my tasty and PCOS-friendly Tomato Avocado Bruschetta, the perfect way to round off our Energizing Starters. A delicious snack that supports your PCOS-friendly journey while also satisfying your palate. Toast to tasty starts and wholesome decisions! Sweet Treats for PCOS

INSTRUCTIONS

1. In a bowl, combine diced cherry tomatoes, diced avocado, minced garlic, and chopped fresh basil. It's a vibrant medley of goodness.
2. Drizzle extra virgin olive oil over the mixture. If you want to kick it up a notch, add a teaspoon of balsamic vinegar. Season with salt and pepper. Give it a gentle toss, letting the flavors mingle.
3. Toast slices of whole-grain or gluten-free bread. This is your PCOS-friendly canvas for the flavorful masterpiece.
4. Spoon the tomato and avocado mix onto the toasted bread slices. It's like crafting tiny, tasty masterpieces.
5. Garnish with a few fresh basil leaves for that final touch of elegance.

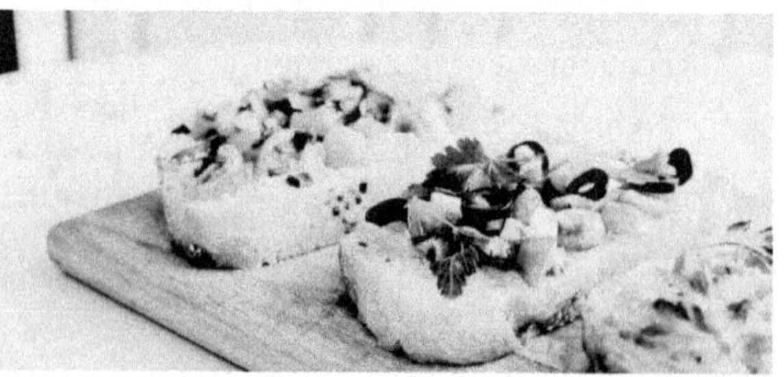

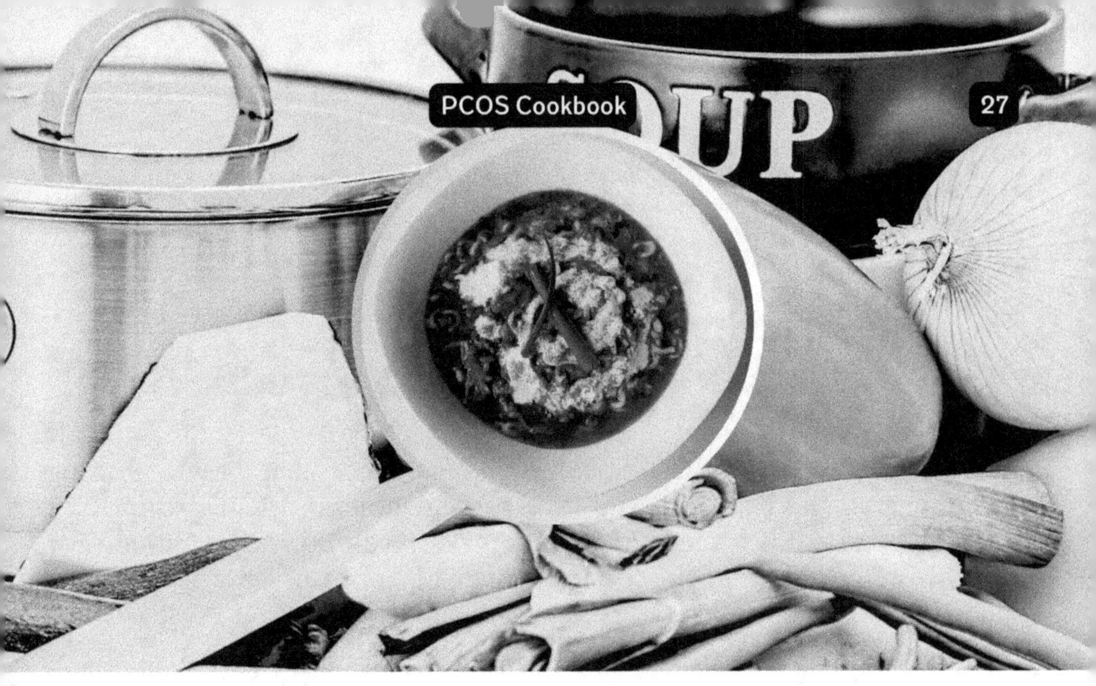

4

A COZY EXPEDITION INTO HEARTY SOUPS

Hi! It's time for Hearty Soups! Get ready to go on a culinary adventure that will warm your entire being, not just your gut! As we delve into this part, comfort, sustenance, and a hint of culinary enchantment are promised with every bite. Come explore five dishes that will soothe your soul: Lentil and Vegetable Soup, Turmeric Chicken Broth, Creamy Pumpkin Soup, Chickpea and Spinach Delight, and Tomato Basil Zoodle Soup to cap it all off. You may be sure that these soups will add heartiness to your table since... They're all suitable for PCOS!

So take out your favorite soup spoon and join me in exploring the heartiness of these delightful dishes. Prepare yourself for an experience that will nourish your body, awaken your sense of taste, and leave you wanting more! 🍲 ✦ A PCOS-Friendly Adventure in Hearty Soup Delights

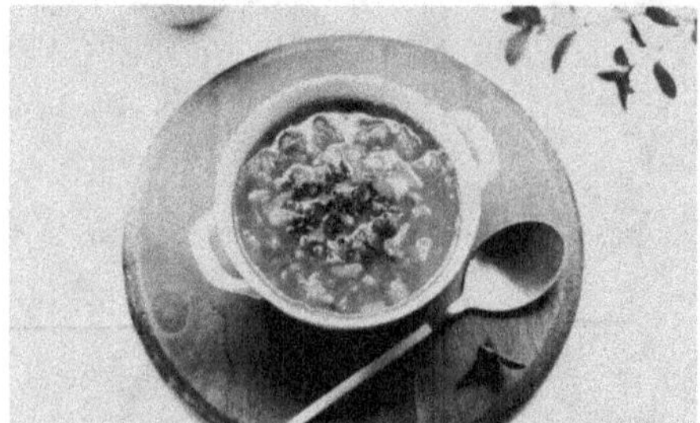

Lentil Veggie: Comfort in a bowl.

Prep ⏰
approx
15 minutes

Cook ⏰
30-40
Minutes

Serves
4-6

Lentil & Vegetable Soup

Greetings, fellow foodies! Speaking of comfort in a bowl, nothing compares to the healthful embrace of vegetable and lentil soup. Not only is it tasty, but it's also a warm, nutrient-rich travel companion for PCOS-friendly eating. So come on over and join us as we prepare a delicious bowl!

INGREDIENTS:

- 1 cup dried lentils (rinsed)
- 2 carrots, diced
- 2 celery stalks, chopped
- 1 onion, finely chopped
- 3 cloves garlic, minced
- 1 can diced tomatoes (14 oz)
- 6 cups vegetable broth
- 1 teaspoon cumin
- 1 teaspoon paprika
- Salt and pepper to taste
- Fresh parsley for garnish

INSTRUCTIONS

1. In a pot, sauté onions and garlic until aromatic. Add carrots and celery, letting them mingle in the flavorful dance.
2. Pour in the vegetable broth and add the dried lentils. Bring it to a gentle boil, then reduce to a simmer.
3. Stir in diced tomatoes, cumin, paprika, salt, and pepper. Let the symphony of flavors simmer until lentils are tender.
4. Ladle up the hearty goodness into bowls, sprinkle some fresh parsley, and savor the warmth!

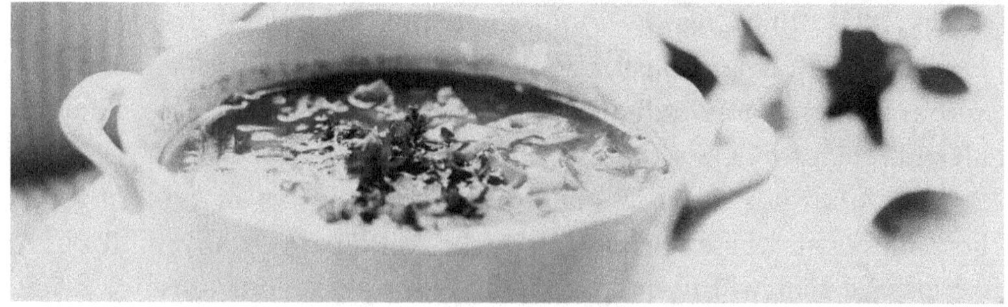

Cheers to delicious, PCOS-friendly Lentil and Vegetable Soup that feels as warm and comfortable as a warm blanket on a winter day. Friends, enjoy the warmth! #PCOSFriendlyCooking #MagicalHeartySoup

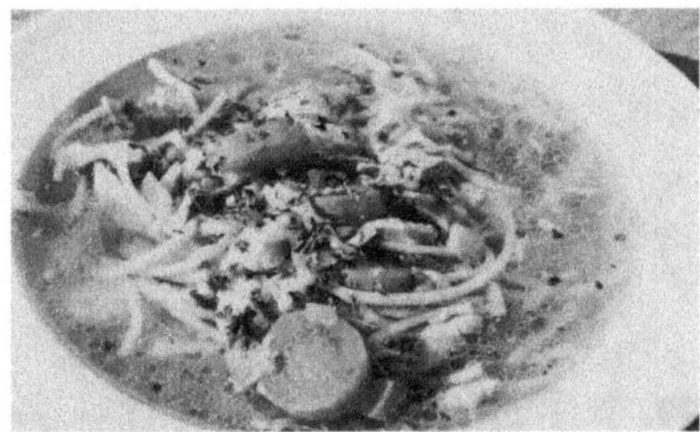

Turmeric Chicken Soup magic. 🍵✦

Turmeric Chicken Soup

Prep ⏰	**Cook** ⏰	**Serves**
15-20 minutes	30 minutes	4-6

Hi there! Prepare to curl up with a bowl of my turmeric chicken soup—a bowl of comfort and well-being. Packed with PCOS-friendly ingredients, it's more than simply a soothing embrace for your taste buds—it makes your meal satisfying and healthful at the same time. Come along on this gastronomic adventure with me!

INGREDIENTS:

- 1 lb boneless, skinless chicken breasts, diced
- 1 cup carrots, sliced
- 1 cup celery, chopped
- 1 cup onion, finely diced
- 3 cloves garlic, minced
- 1 tablespoon fresh turmeric, grated
- 1 teaspoon ground ginger
- 6 cups chicken broth (low-sodium)
- 1 cup kale, chopped
- 1 cup zucchini, diced
- Salt and pepper to taste
- Fresh parsley for garnish

Here it is, my recipe for Turmeric Chicken Soup! A bowlful of cozy goodness enhanced with the health benefits of turmeric, created to make your journey toward wellness a tasty journey. Savor the comforting warmth! #TurmericChickenSoup 🍵✦

INSTRUCTIONS

1. In a large pot over medium heat, sauté diced chicken until browned. Remove and set aside.
2. In the same pot, add a bit of olive oil if needed and sauté carrots, celery, and onion until softened.
3. Stir in minced garlic, grated turmeric, and ground ginger. Let the aromatic symphony unfold for a minute.
4. Pour in chicken broth and bring the mixture to a gentle boil.
5. Add the browned chicken back to the pot and simmer for about 15–20 minutes until the chicken is cooked through.
6. Toss in kale and zucchini, letting them cook for an additional 5 minutes.
7. Season with salt and pepper to suit your taste.
8. Ladle the golden goodness into bowls, garnish with fresh parsley, and savor the comforting delight!

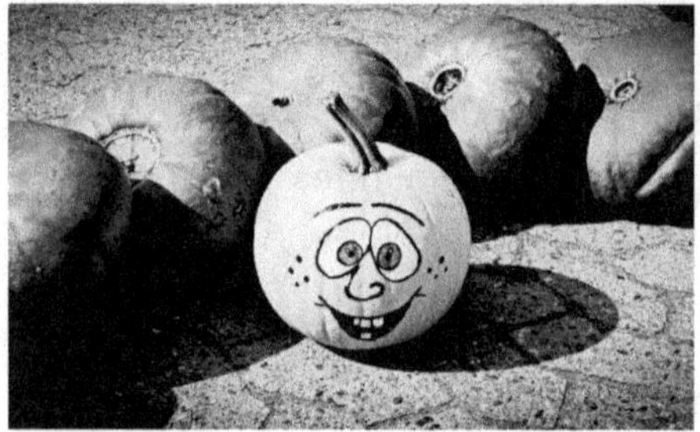

Creamy Pumpkin Soup

Prep ⏰	**Cook** ⏱	**Serves**
approx 15 minutes	25-30 minutes	4-6

Hi! Today I'm sharing a beloved recipe with you, Creamy Pumpkin Soup, which is like a warm embrace in a bowl. It's a PCOS-friendly treat that delivers the comforting tastes of fall to your table, so it's not only about the thick, velvety texture. Let's savor the delicious creaminess!

INGREDIENTS:

- 1 medium-sized pumpkin, peeled and diced
- 1 onion, chopped
- 2 carrots, roughly chopped
- 3 cloves garlic, minced
- 1 teaspoon ground cinnamon
- 1/2 teaspoon nutmeg
- 4 cups vegetable broth
- 1 cup coconut milk
- Salt and pepper to taste
- Pumpkin seeds for garnish

INSTRUCTIONS

1. In a pot, sauté onions and garlic until golden. Add diced pumpkin and carrots, letting them mingle in the flavorful dance.
2. Sprinkle in ground cinnamon and nutmeg, infusing those cozy fall vibes. Pour in vegetable broth, bringing everything to a gentle simmer.
3. Let it simmer until the pumpkin and carrots are tender – about 20-25 minutes. Grab your trusty blender and blend until smooth.
4. Pour in the creamy coconut milk, stirring until the soup reaches the perfect velvety consistency. Season with salt and pepper, adjusting to your taste.
5. Ladle this golden elixir into bowls, and for that extra touch, sprinkle pumpkin seeds on top.

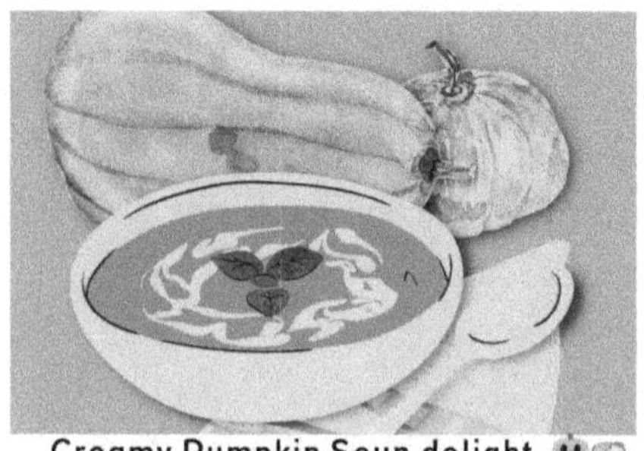

Creamy Pumpkin Soup delight. 🎃🥣

There you have it: my recipe for Creamy Pumpkin Soup, a hearty and warming dish that is suitable for those with PCOS. My friends, savor this bowl of luscious comfort! 🎃🥣
#VegetarianCooking #MagicalPumpkin

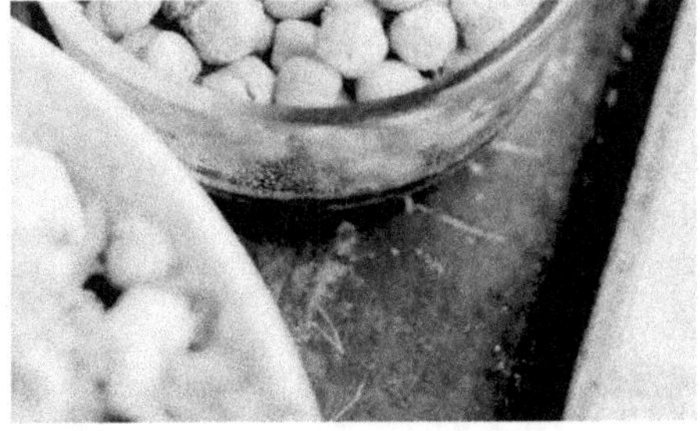

Prep ⏰	Cook ⏰	Serves
approx 15 minutes	about 20 minutes	4-6

Chickpea & Spinach Delight

Greetings, fellow cooks! I'm revealing one of my all-time favorite PCOS-friendly recipes today, or rather, I'm spilling the beans, as it were. My Chickpea and Spinach Delight is waiting for you to curl up with it. It's a tasty and nutritious combination of flavors that is hearty and satisfying. Let's get started on the deliciousness!

INGREDIENTS:

- 1 can chickpeas, drained and rinsed
- 1 onion, finely chopped
- 3 cloves garlic, minced
- 1 teaspoon cumin
- 1 teaspoon paprika
- 4 cups vegetable broth
- 1 can diced tomatoes
- 4 cups fresh spinach leaves
- Salt and pepper to taste
- Fresh lemon wedges for serving

INSTRUCTIONS

1. In a pot, sauté the finely chopped onion and minced garlic until they dance into golden perfection.
2. Sprinkle in cumin and paprika, letting those aromatic spices mingle with the veggies.
3. Add the drained chickpeas, vegetable broth, and diced tomatoes to the pot. Bring this flavorful party to a simmer.
4. Toss in the fresh spinach leaves, letting them wilt into the mix. Season with salt and pepper, adjusting to your liking.
5. Let the soup simmer for about 15-20 minutes, allowing all those fantastic flavors to intermingle.
6. Ladle this delightful concoction into bowls and serve with a squeeze of fresh lemon for that extra zing.

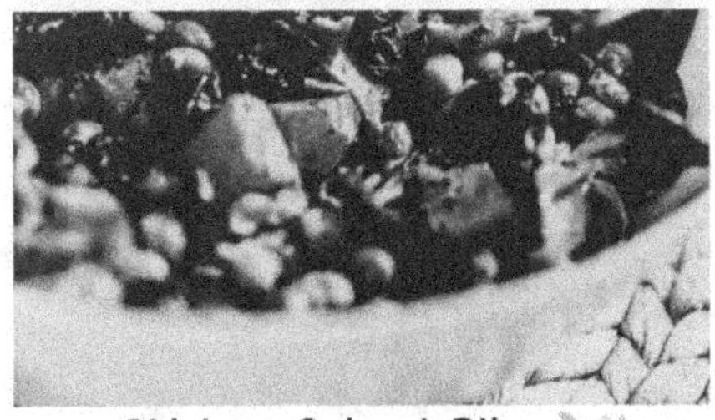

Chickpea Spinach Bliss. 🍸

This is my recipe for Chickpea and Spinach Delight, a flavorful and nutritious dish that is suitable for people with PCOS. Enjoy, folks, this dish of goodness! 🍵🍸 #PCOSFriendlyCooking #DeliciousChickpea Spinach

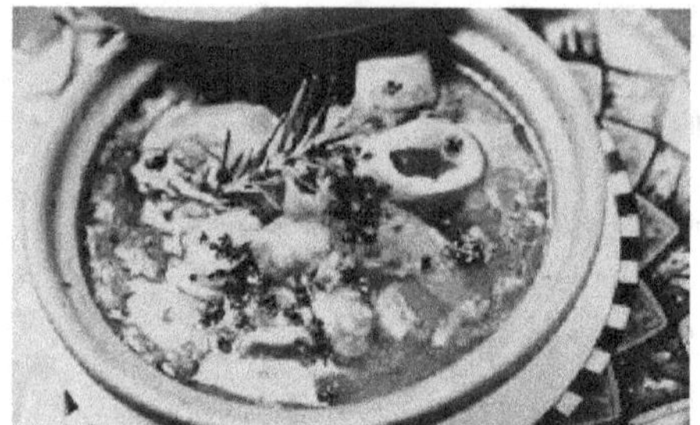

Tomato Basil Zoodle bliss.

Prep ⏰	Cook ⏰	Serves
approx 15 minutes	about 15 minutes	4-6

Tomato Basil Zoodle

Hi there! I'm bringing out the colorful flavors of my favorite comfort food that works for PCOS, tomato basil zoodle soup, today. This delicious bowl not only pleases your palate but also fits in with a PCOS-aware way of living. Let's go on a voyage of delicious adventure!

INGREDIENTS:

- 4 medium-sized zucchinis, spiralized into zoodles
- 1 onion, finely chopped
- 3 cloves garlic, minced
- 1 can crushed tomatoes
- 4 cups vegetable broth
- 1 teaspoon dried basil
- 1 teaspoon dried oregano
- Salt and pepper to taste
- Fresh basil leaves for garnish
- Parmesan cheese (optional)

INSTRUCTIONS

1. In a pot, sauté the finely chopped onion and minced garlic until they become a golden symphony of flavor.
2. Add the spiralized zucchini to the pot, letting them mingle with the aromatic dance of onions and garlic.
3. Pour in the crushed tomatoes and vegetable broth, bringing this flavorful fiesta to a simmer.
4. Season with dried basil, oregano, salt, and pepper, letting the herbs infuse their magic into the soup.
5. Let the zoodles simmer until tender, usually around 8-10 minutes.
6. Ladle this delightful creation into bowls, garnishing with fresh basil leaves and a sprinkle of Parmesan if you fancy.

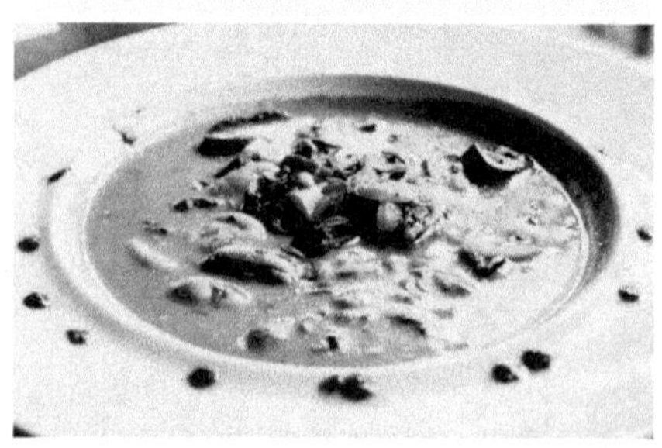

Here it is: my delicious and nutritious Tomato Basil Zoodle Soup, a comforting dish that is suitable for those with PCOS. Enjoy the wonderful adventure as you dive into this bowl of delight! #VeganFriendlyCooking #Magical Zoodle Soup

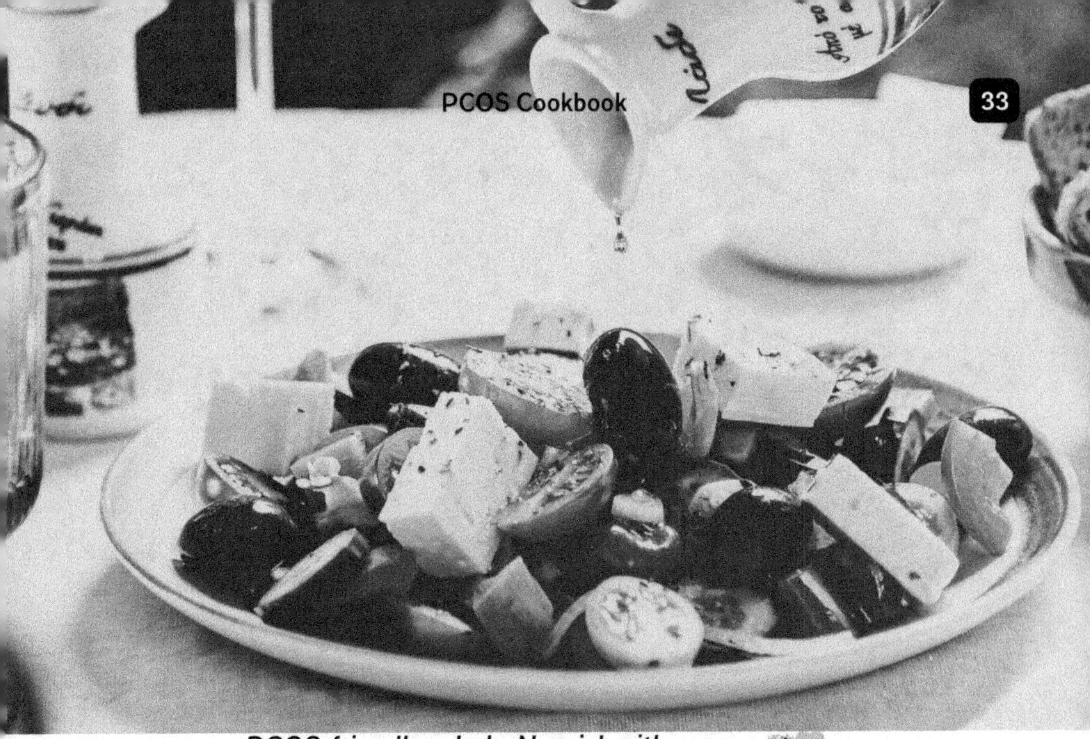

PCOS-friendly salads: Nourish with greens.

5

VIBRANT PCOS-FRIENDLY SALADS

Hello, fans of salads! I am going to take you on a tour through a colorful, PCOS-friendly salad garden. These bowls are designed to complement a well-being-promoting lifestyle in addition to being vibrantly colored. Now let's enjoy the crisp freshness of some of my favorite salads: Avocado Chickpea Delight, Roasted Beet with Goat Cheese, Quinoa Power Salad, Citrus Shrimp, and Kale and Cranberry. A symphony of flavors and minerals is about to unfold! Happy #PCOSSaladAdventure

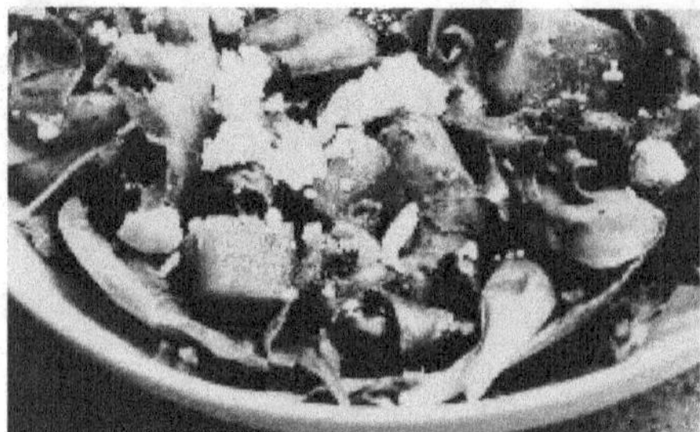

A salad sensation!

Kale & Cranberry Salad

Fans of salads, rejoice! I'm sharing the wonderful story behind my favorite PCOS-friendly dish, kale and cranberry salad, today. In addition to adding a pop of color to your table, this dish is a great fit for a PCOS-aware way of living. Get ready to indulge in deliciousness!

Prep ⏰
15 minutes

Cook ⏰
0 minutes

Serves
4

INGREDIENTS:

- 6 cups fresh kale, stems removed and chopped
- 1 cup dried cranberries
- 1/2 cup walnuts, chopped
- 1/4 cup feta cheese, crumbled
- 1 apple, thinly sliced
- 1/4 cup extra virgin olive oil
- 2 tablespoons balsamic vinegar
- 1 tablespoon maple syrup
- Salt and pepper to taste

INSTRUCTIONS

1. In a large bowl, massage the kale with olive oil for a couple of minutes until it becomes tender.
2. Toss in the dried cranberries, chopped walnuts, crumbled feta, and the thinly sliced apple, creating a colorful canvas of flavors.
3. In a small bowl, whisk together the balsamic vinegar, maple syrup, salt, and pepper, creating the perfect dressing.
4. Drizzle the dressing over the salad, ensuring every leaf gets a taste of the flavorful harmony.
5. Toss the salad gently, making sure the dressing coats every ingredient lovingly.
6. Serve this vibrant bowl of goodness and savor the PCOS-friendly crunch!

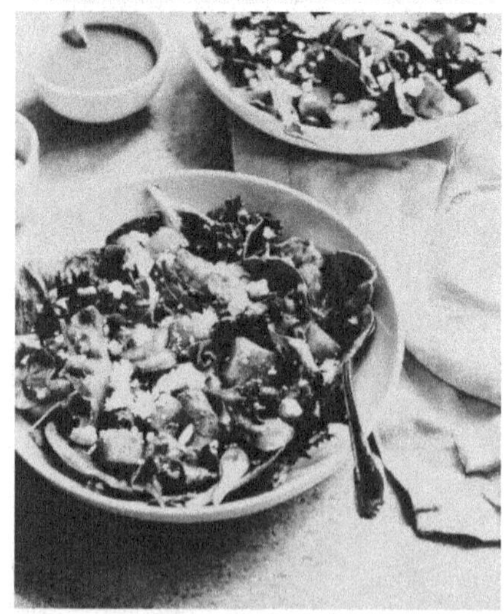

That's my Kale and Cranberry Salad, a delicious and nutritious dish that is also PCOS-friendly. Let's savor the tastes and appreciate the crunch of goodness! 🍴 🫐
#PCOSSaladMagic

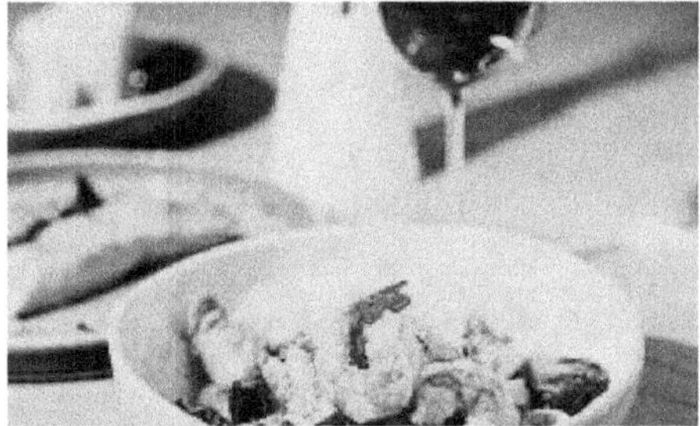

Citrus Shrimp Salad: Fresh & zesty!

Prep ⏰	Cook ⏰	Serves
20 minutes	Speedy shrimp perfection (5 minutes)	4

Citrus Shrimp Salad

Dear salad fans, I'm excited to share one of my all-time faves on this page: citrus shrimp salad. This salad is a wonderful celebration of freshness, full of brilliant tastes and deliciousness that is suitable for those with PCOS. Now let's get started on the recipe and make a tasty bowl!

INGREDIENTS:

- 1 lb shrimp, peeled and deveined
- 4 cups mixed salad greens
- 1 grapefruit, segmented
- 1 orange, segmented
- 1 avocado, sliced
- 1/4 cup red onion, thinly sliced
- 2 tablespoons fresh cilantro, chopped
- 2 tablespoons olive oil
- 1 tablespoon honey
- 1 tablespoon lime juice
- Salt and pepper to taste

INSTRUCTIONS

1. Season the shrimp with salt and pepper. In a pan over medium heat, cook the shrimp until pink and opaque. Set aside.
2. In a large bowl, combine the mixed salad greens, grapefruit segments, orange segments, avocado slices, red onion, and cilantro.
3. For the dressing, whisk together olive oil, honey, lime juice, salt, and pepper. Drizzle it over the salad.
4. Gently toss the salad to ensure every ingredient gets a taste of that zesty dressing.
5. Top the salad with the cooked shrimp, arranging them like the crowning jewels.
6. Serve this citrus-infused masterpiece and enjoy the burst of flavors!

There you have it: my Citrus Shrimp Salad, which adds a marine flavor to your salad bowl and is suitable for those with PCOS. Savor each bright taste as you dive into freshness!
PCOSSaladMagic

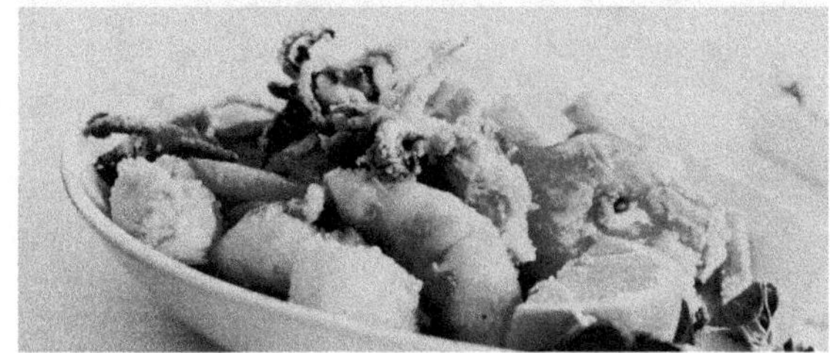

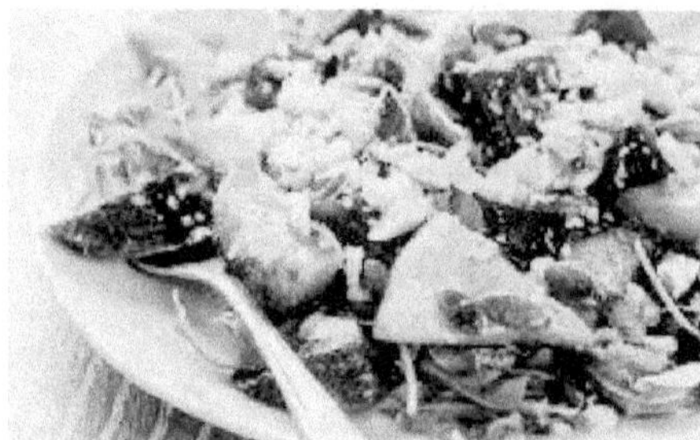

A vibrant medley. 🥗🍴

Prep ⏰	Cook ⏰	Serves
10 minutes	25-30 minutes	4

Roasted Beet & Goat Cheese Salad

Hi! With my Roasted Beet & Goat Cheese Salad, I'm bringing a rainbow of colors and flavors to your plate. This delicious dessert that is suitable for people with PCOS is not only gorgeous to look at but also delicious. Let's go on a colorful, delicious adventure!

INGREDIENTS:

- 3 medium-sized beets, peeled and cubed
- 4 cups mixed salad greens
- 1/2 cup goat cheese, crumbled
- 1/4 cup walnuts, toasted
- 1/4 cup balsamic vinaigrette
- 2 tablespoons olive oil
- Salt and pepper to taste

Here it is: my Roasted Beet & Goat Cheese Salad, a visually pleasing and aesthetically pleasing mix that is suitable for those with PCOS. Savor the vibrant voyage! 🌈🥗 #PCOSSaladMagic

INSTRUCTIONS

1. Preheat your oven to 400°F (200°C).
2. Toss the cubed beets with olive oil, salt, and pepper. Roast them in the preheated oven for about 25-30 minutes or until they're tender and slightly caramelized.
3. In a large bowl, combine the mixed salad greens, crumbled goat cheese, and toasted walnuts.
4. Once the beets are roasted to perfection, let them cool slightly before adding them to the salad.
5. Drizzle the balsamic vinaigrette over the salad and give it a gentle toss to coat all the ingredients.
6. Serve this vibrant masterpiece on your favorite plate and get ready to indulge in a symphony of colors and flavors!

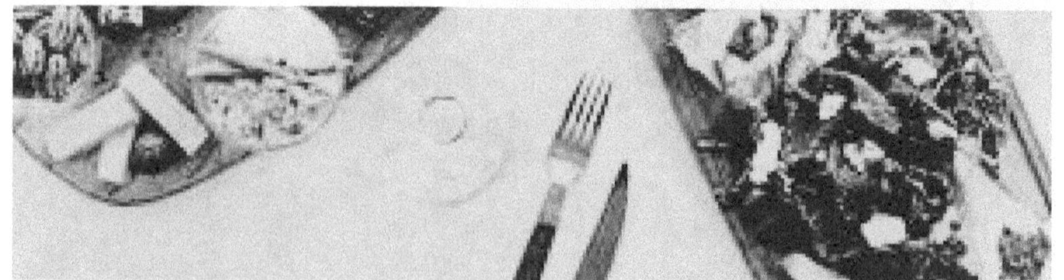

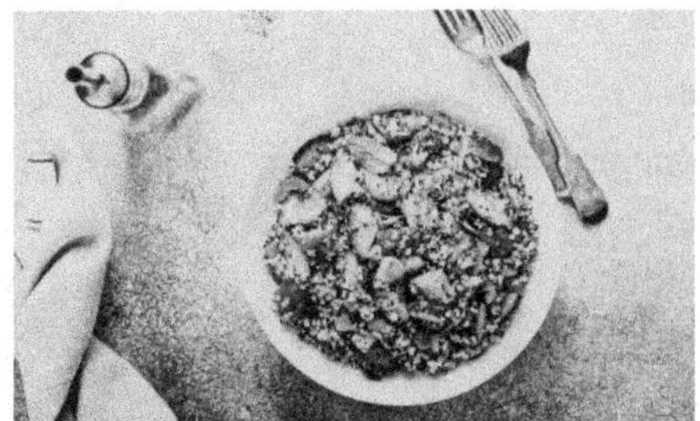

Fuel for greatness.

Prep ⏰	Cook ⏰	Serves
15 minutes	15 minutes	4

Quinoa Power Salad

Hi there! Prepare to fuel your day with my Quinoa Power Salad, a bowl full of goodness. This PCOS-friendly recipe is more than just a salad because to its abundance of nutrient-rich vegetables; it's a celebration of flavors and well-being. Now let's get started!

INGREDIENTS:

- 1 cup quinoa, rinsed
- 2 cups water or vegetable broth
- 1 cup cherry tomatoes, halved
- 1 cucumber, diced
- 1/2 cup red bell pepper, chopped
- 1/4 cup red onion, finely diced
- 1/4 cup feta cheese, crumbled
- 1/4 cup Kalamata olives, sliced
- 1/4 cup fresh parsley, chopped

INSTRUCTIONS

1. In a saucepan, combine quinoa and water or vegetable broth. Bring it to a boil, then reduce the heat, cover, and simmer for about 15 minutes or until quinoa is cooked and water is absorbed. Fluff with a fork and let it cool.
2. In a large bowl, mix together the cooked quinoa, cherry tomatoes, cucumber, red bell pepper, red onion, feta cheese, Kalamata olives, and fresh parsley.
3. Toss the salad with your favorite dressing or a simple olive oil and lemon vinaigrette.
4. Serve it up in your favorite bowl and relish the power-packed goodness!

Here it is: my Quinoa Power Salad, a delicious and healthy dish that is suitable for people with PCOS and will satisfy your taste buds and body. Savor the colorful road towards better health!

#PCOSSaladPower

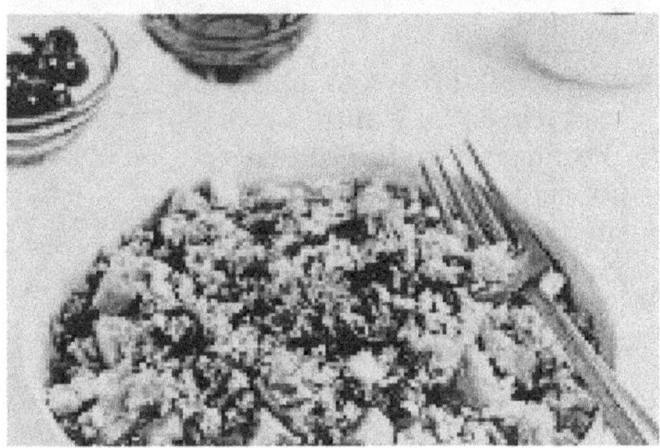

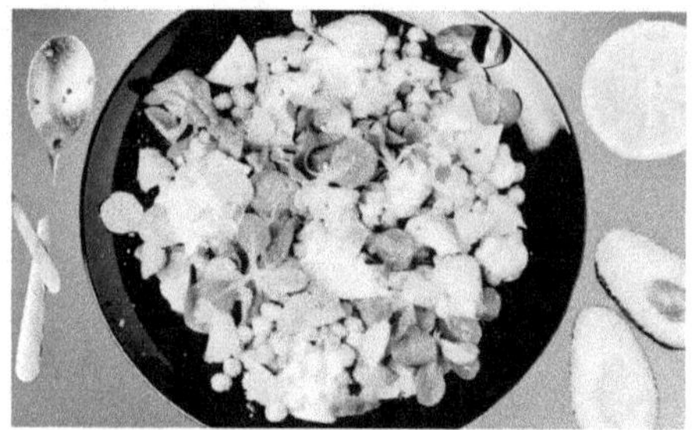

Simple bliss in every bite. 🥑🍸

Prep ⏰	Cook ⏰	Serves
15 minutes	0 minutes	2

Avocado Chickpea Delight

Salads should be bright and colorful, so say goodbye to boring ones! Not only is my Avocado Chickpea Delight Salad a delicious alternative, but it's also a nutritious choice made with PCOS-friendly foods to make your journey to wellness enjoyable.

INGREDIENTS:

- 2 ripe avocados, diced
- 1 can (15 oz) chickpeas, drained and rinsed
- 1 cup cherry tomatoes, halved
- 1 cucumber, peeled and diced
- 1/4 cup red onion, finely chopped
- 1/4 cup fresh cilantro, chopped
- Juice of 1 lemon
- 2 tablespoons extra virgin olive oil
- Salt and pepper to taste

INSTRUCTIONS

1. In a large mixing bowl, combine diced avocados, chickpeas, cherry tomatoes, cucumber, red onion, and fresh cilantro.
2. Drizzle the lemon juice and extra virgin olive oil over the salad ingredients.
3. Gently toss the salad to ensure all ingredients are well coated with the dressing.
4. Season with salt and pepper according to your taste preferences.
5. Chill in the refrigerator for about 15-20 minutes to let the flavors mingle.
6. Serve in your favorite salad bowl and savor the delightful goodness!

That's my Avocado Chickpea Delight Salad for you. This salad will leave you wanting more because it's so full of tastes, nutrients, and goodness that's suitable for those with PCOS. Savor this enjoyable path to better health! 🥑🥑
#VegetableChickpeaDelicious

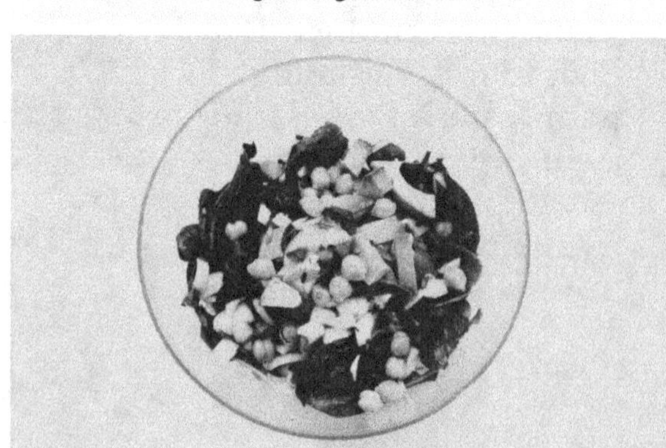

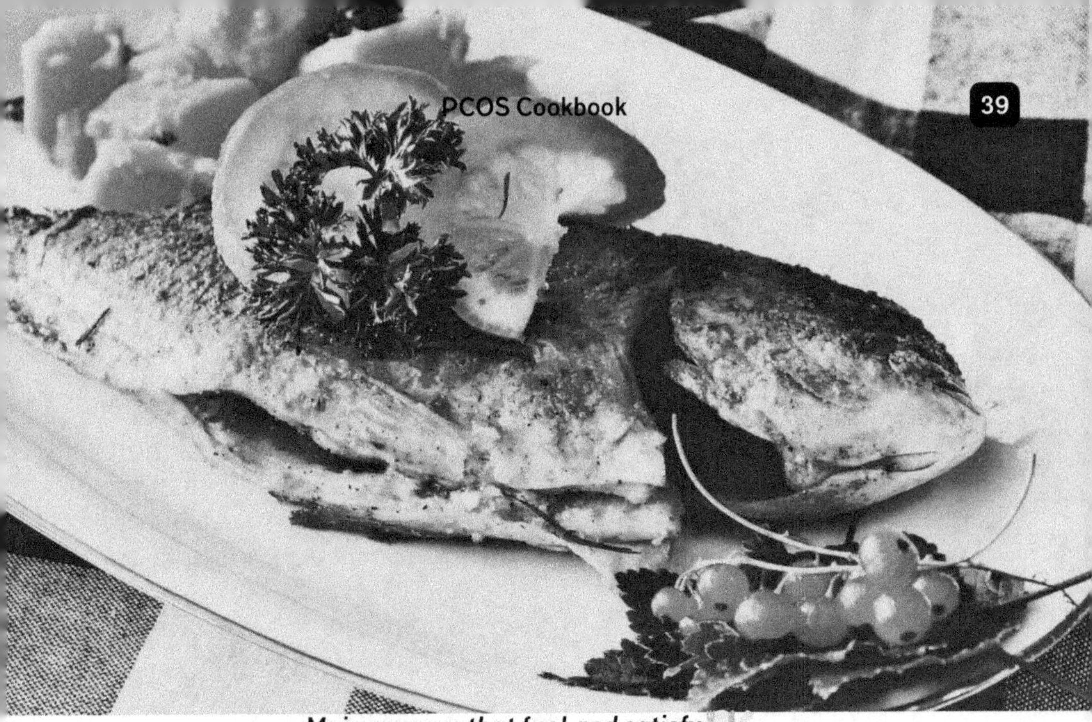

Main courses that fuel and satisfy

6

LEAN PROTEIN MAIN COURSES

Hello, food enthusiasts! Welcome to the heart of your balanced meals – my Lean Protein Main Courses: . Grilled Salmon with Lemon Dill Sauce, Turkey and Quinoa Stuffed Peppers, Tofu Stir-Fry with Broccoli, Lemon Herb Baked Chicken, and Chickpea and Spinach Curry.

These recipes aren't just about the flavors; they're designed to keep your PCOS-friendly lifestyle in check. Let's dive into this section where every bite is a step toward nourishing your well-being.

Get ready to savor the perfect balance of protein-packed goodness. Let the culinary adventure begin! #LeanProteinDelights

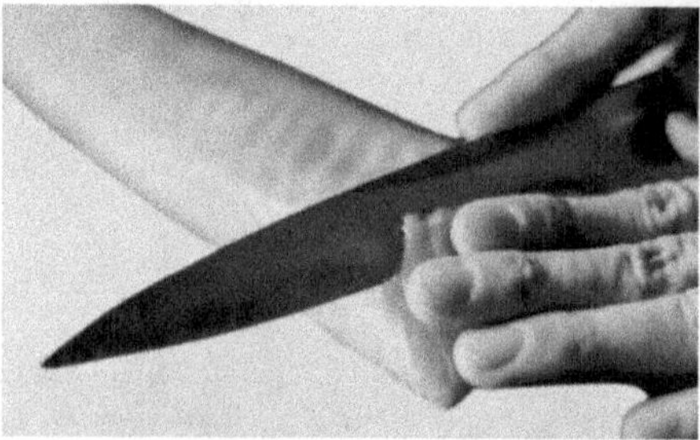

Prep ⏰
10 minutes

Cook ⏰
10 minutes

Serves
4

Grilled Salmon with Lemon Dill Sauce

Ahoy, seafood lovers! This recipe for Grilled Salmon with Lemon Dill Sauce is more than simply a meal; it's a taste adventure. This recipe is designed to be PCOS-friendly and is full of goodies with omega-3 fatty acids. Come along for a delicious seafood journey as we light up the grill!

INGREDIENTS:

- 5 fillets of salmon
- Add salt and pepper to taste.
- 2 teaspoons of olive oil
- 2 teaspoons finely chopped fresh dill
- 1 lemon's zest
- Half a lemon's juice

There you have it: a taste-bud feast that will also help your PCOS-friendly menu. Savor the deliciously delectable Grilled Salmon with Lemon Dill Sauce! #SalmonSensation

INSTRUCTIONS

1. Preheat your grill to medium-high heat.
2. Add salt and pepper to the salmon fillets for seasoning.
3. To make the marinade, combine olive oil, lemon zest, lemon juice, and chopped dill in a small bowl.
4. Apply a thick coating of marinade to the salmon fillets.
5. The salmon should flake easily when tested with a fork, which takes around 4–5 minutes on each side.
6. Drizzle an additional portion of lemon-dill sauce over your salmon before serving.

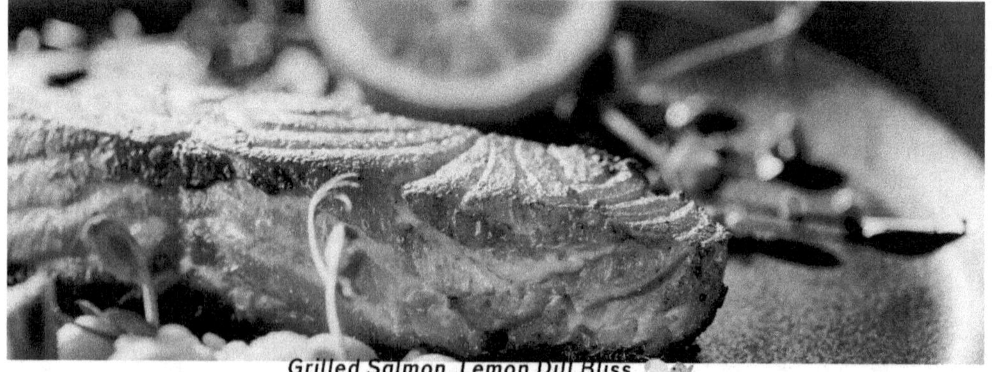

Grilled Salmon, Lemon Dill Bliss.

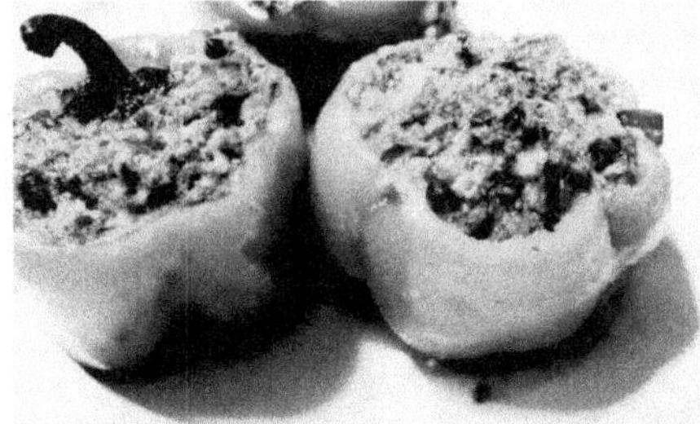

A taste-packed twist.

| **Prep** ⏰ | **Cook** ⏰ | **Serves** |
| 20 minutes | 35-40 minutes | 4 |

Turkey & Quinoa Stuffed Peppers

All set to host a fiesta for dinner? These colorful, healthy, and perfectly suited for PCOS turkey and quinoa stuffed peppers are more than just a visual treat. Let's embark on a delectable nutrient and flavor journey!

INGREDIENTS:

- 4 large bell peppers, cut in half and seeded; one pound of minced turkey 1 cup of cooked quinoa; and
- 1 cup of rinsed and drained black beans
- 1 cup of corn kernels, either fresh or frozen
- 1 cup of chopped tomatoes
- 1 cup of shredded cheese (either cheddar or another type of cheese of your choosing)
- 1 teaspoon of ground cumin
- 1 teaspoon of chili powder
- Add salt and pepper to taste
- Garnish with fresh cilantro

INSTRUCTIONS

1. Turn the oven on to 375°F, or 190°C.
2. Brown the ground turkey in a pan over medium heat.
3. The cooked turkey, cooked quinoa, black beans, corn, diced tomatoes, cumin, chili powder, salt, and pepper should all be combined in a big mixing bowl.
4. In each half of a bell pepper, stuff the turkey-quinoa mixture.
5. Spoon the remaining cheese over the stuffed peppers in a baking tray.
6. Bake the dish for 25 to 30 minutes with the foil covering it. When the cheese is bubbling, remove the top and bake for a further five to ten minutes.
7. Add fresh cilantro as a garnish before serving.

Voila! Your Turkey and Quinoa Stuffed Peppers are ready to steal the spotlight at your dinner table. Dive into this PCOS-friendly delight that's as nutritious as it is delicious!
#StuffedPepperJoy

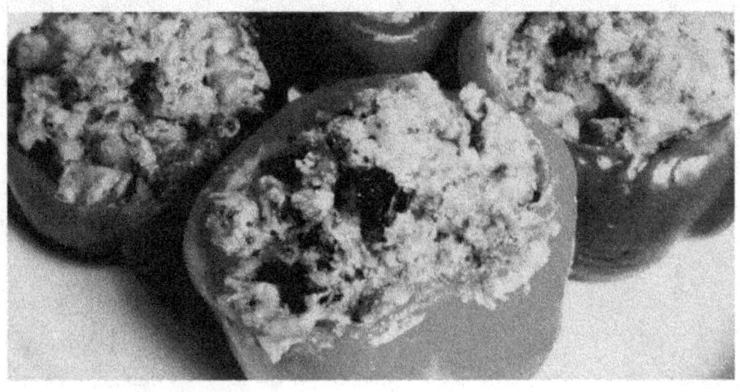

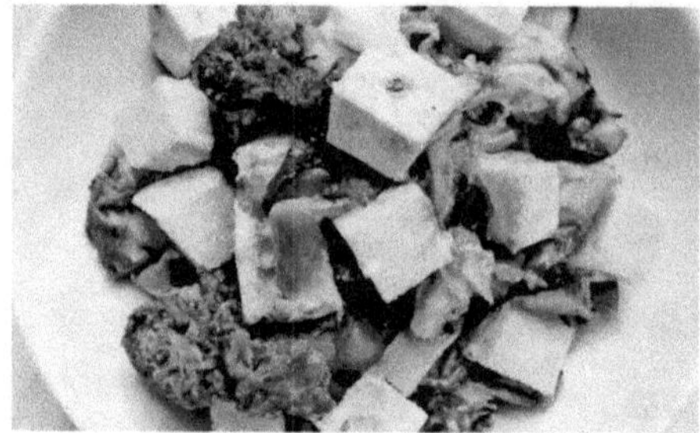

T&B Stir-Fry: Quick and tasty.

Prep ⏰
15 minutes

Cook ⏰
15 minutes

Serves
4

Tofu Stir-Fry with Broccoli

Are you prepared to up your supper game with a taste explosion? Not only is this tofu stir-fry with broccoli a culinary delight, but it's also a PCOS-friendly powerhouse. Let's go on an adventure to make a tasty and nourishing dish!

INGREDIENTS:

- 1 block extra-firm tofu, pressed and cubed
- 2 cups broccoli florets
- 1 bell pepper, thinly sliced
- 1 carrot, julienned
- 1 cup snap peas, ends trimmed
- 3 tablespoons soy sauce
- 2 tablespoons hoisin sauce
- 1 tablespoon sesame oil
- 1 tablespoon rice vinegar
- 2 cloves garlic, minced
- 1 teaspoon fresh ginger, grated
- 2 tablespoons vegetable oil
- Sesame seeds for garnish (optional)
- Green onions for garnish, sliced

INSTRUCTIONS

1. In a bowl, whisk together soy sauce, hoisin sauce, sesame oil, and rice vinegar to create the sauce.
2. Heat vegetable oil in a wok or large skillet over medium-high heat.
3. Add tofu cubes and stir-fry until golden brown on all sides. Remove tofu from the wok and set aside.
4. In the same wok, stir-fry broccoli, bell pepper, carrot, snap peas, garlic, and ginger until vegetables are tender-crisp.
5. Add the cooked tofu back to the wok and pour the sauce over the mixture. Toss everything together until well coated.
6. Garnish with sesame seeds and sliced green onions.

Here you have it: a flavorful and fulfilling Tofu Stir-Fry with Broccoli that can help you achieve your PCOS control objectives while also pleasing your palate. Prepare to enjoy every delicious bite! #StirFryDelight

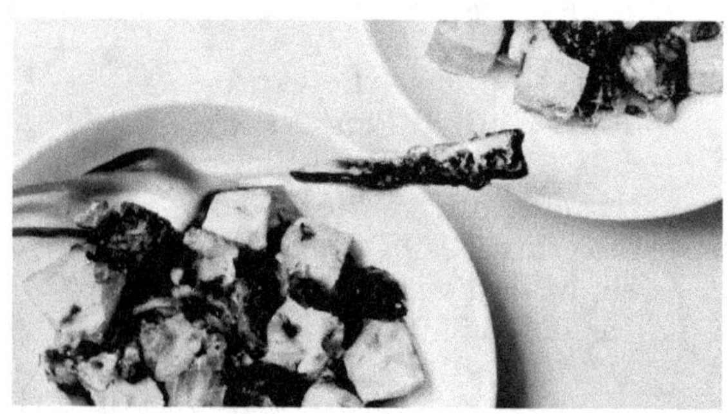

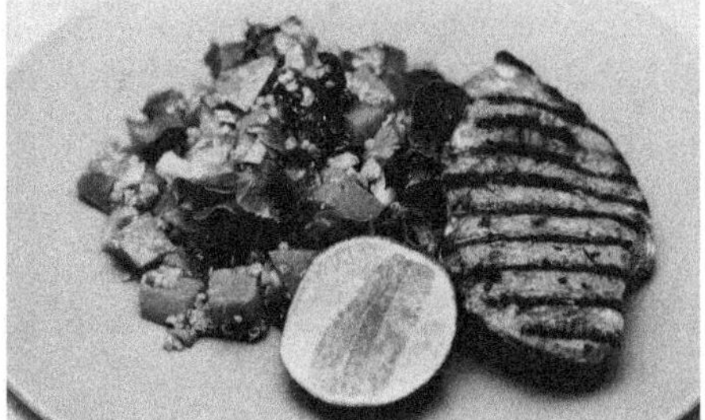

Lemon Herb Chicken: Simply zesty.

Prep ⏰	Cook ⏰	Serves
10 minutes	25-30 minutes	4

Lemon Herb Baked Chicken

Boost your supper experience with a spicy flavor explosion! Not only is this Lemon Herb Baked Chicken delicious, but it's also a PCOS-friendly joy. Let's explore the healthful properties of citrus and herbs for a lunch!

INGREDIENTS:

- 2 tablespoons olive oil
- 2 minced garlic cloves
- 1 teaspoon each of dried oregano, thyme, and rosemary
- 4 skinless and boneless chicken breasts
- 1 zesty lemon
- Add pepper and salt for seasoning. Add fresh parsley as a garnish.

INSTRUCTIONS

1. Preheat the oven to 375°F, or 190°C.
2. In a small bowl, mix together the lemon juice, zest, olive oil, minced garlic, oregano, thyme, rosemary, salt, and pepper.
3. Transfer the chicken breasts to a roasting tray. Make sure to properly coat each piece of chicken with the lemon-herb mixture before covering it.
4. Bake in the preheated oven for 25 to 30 minutes, or until the internal temperature reaches 165°F (74°C).
5. Add some fresh parsley as a garnish before serving.

You're not just enjoying a delicious dinner when you bite into this Lemon Herb Baked Chicken—you're also embracing a PCOS-friendly alternative that tastes good and nourishes. Savor the tastes! #HerbInfusionMagic

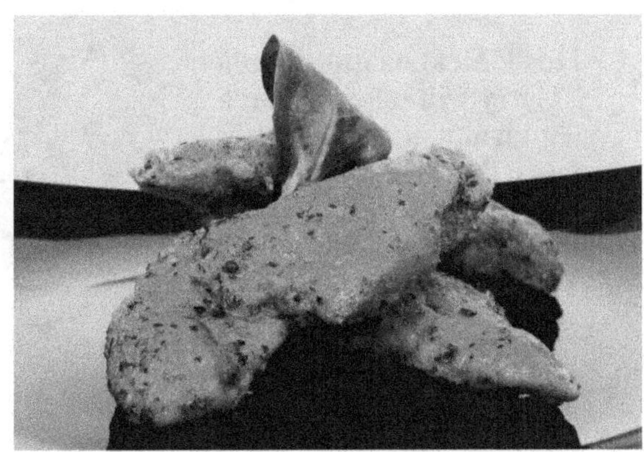

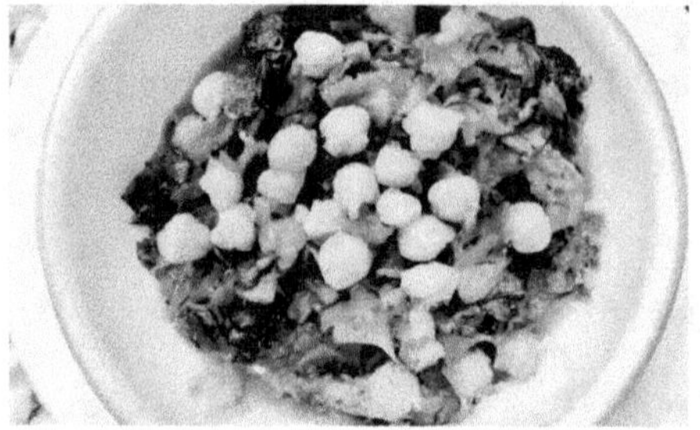

Chickpea Spinach Curry: Pure delight

Prep ⏰
15 minutes

Cook ⏰
20 minutes

Serves
4

Chickpea & Spinach Curry Delight

Do you have a need for a tasty, yet PCOS-friendly, soothing curry? There's nowhere else to look! A healthy combination of flavors and nutrients, this curry with chickpeas and spinach is a great addition to your dish collection.

INGREDIENTS:

- 2 cans (15 oz each) chickpeas, drained and rinsed
- 1 onion, finely chopped
- 3 tomatoes, diced
- 2 cups fresh spinach
- 3 cloves garlic, minced
- 1-inch ginger, grated
- 1 can (14 oz) coconut milk
- 2 tablespoons curry powder
- 1 teaspoon cumin
- 1 teaspoon turmeric
- Salt and pepper to taste
- 2 tablespoons cooking oil
- Fresh cilantro for garnish

INSTRUCTIONS

1. In a pan, heat oil over medium heat. Add chopped onions and cook until golden brown.
2. Stir in garlic and ginger, sautéing for a minute until fragrant.
3. Add curry powder, cumin, and turmeric. Mix well to coat the onions evenly.
4. Pour in diced tomatoes and cook until they soften, forming a thick base.
5. Add chickpeas, spinach, and coconut milk. Season with salt and pepper. Simmer for 15-20 minutes.
6. Garnish with fresh cilantro before serving.

This Chickpea and Spinach Curry will take you on a gourmet adventure. It's more than simply a meal— it's a celebration on your plate, full of health and flavor. Savor each healthy spoonful! 🥄
#CurryCravingHappy

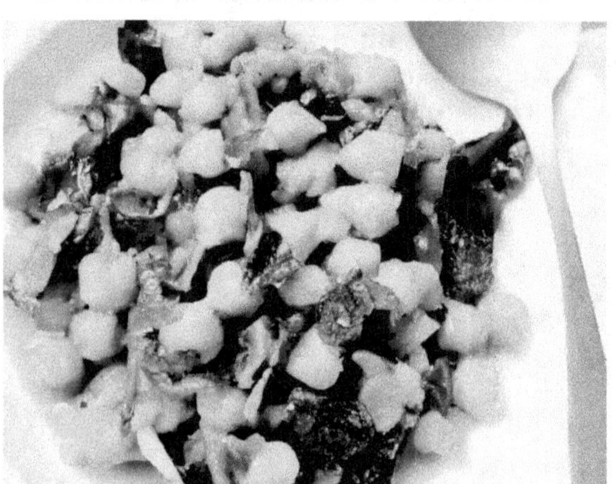

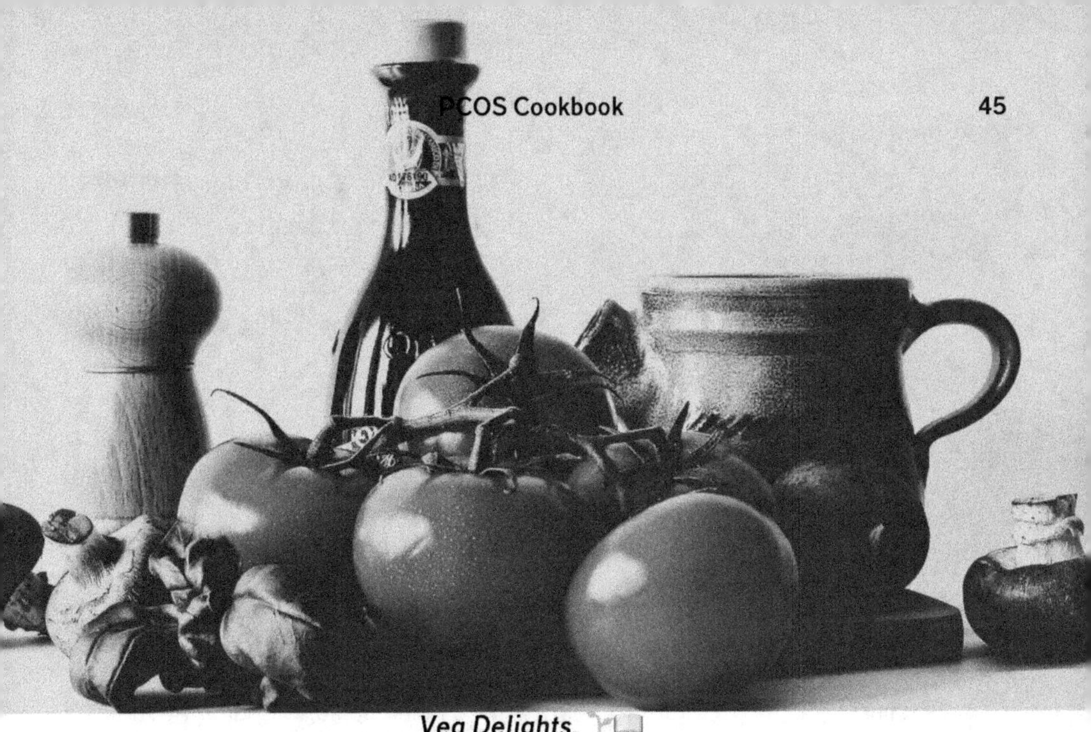

Veg Delights.

7
VEGETARIAN DELIGHTS

Welcome to a delightful journey through my Vegetarian Delights section. I've curated a collection of vibrant and satisfying dishes that celebrate the goodness of plant-based ingredients. Join me in savoring the refreshing Zucchini Noodles with Pesto, the hearty Cauliflower and Chickpea Curry, the comforting Eggplant Lasagna, the wholesome Spinach & Feta Stuffed Portobello Mushrooms, and the flavorful Quinoa & Roasted Vegetable Buddha Bowl.

Each dish is carefully crafted to tantalize your taste buds while being mindful of PCOS-friendly ingredients. Let's dive into the world of wholesome and flavorful vegetarian options that make every meal a celebration of nourishing goodness. #VegetarianJoy

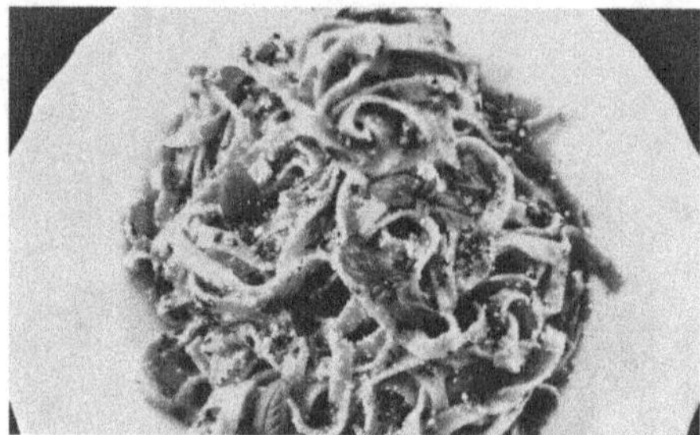

Zucchini Noodles, Pesto Bliss.

Prep ⏰
15 minutes

Cook ⏰
0 minutes

Serves
2-3

Zucchini Noodles with Pesto

Oh, my pesto-crusted zucchini noodles are a delicious way to satiate your palate without going too far in the PCOS direction. Together, let's embark on this gastronomic adventure!

INGREDIENTS:

- 4 spiralized medium-sized zucchini
- 1 cup of freshl basil leaves
- 1/4 cup pine nuts
- 1/3 cup shredded Parmesan cheese
- 2 minced garlic cloves
- 1/2 cup of extra virgin olive oil
- Season with salt and pepper
- Garnish with cherry tomatoes (optional)

Enjoy this light and PCOS-friendly recipe that combines the flavor of homemade pesto with the health of zucchini. To enhance your gourmet experience, try serving it with grilled chicken or a side dish of quinoa for a heartier meal. Cheers to guilt-free decadence!

INSTRUCTIONS

1. Start by spiralizing the zucchinis into strands that resemble noodles. Put them in a big basin and set away.
2. Get the Pesto Sauce Ready: Minced garlic, pine nuts, basil, and Parmesan cheese should all be combined in a food processor. Pulse until chopped finely. Add olive oil little by little, pulsing until smooth consistency is reached. Add pepper and salt for seasoning.
3. Combine Pesto and Zoodles: Cover the zucchini noodles with the pesto sauce. Gently toss everything together, making sure the noodles get coated all over in that bright green goodness.
4. It's time to serve your pesto zucchini noodles! Add some cherry tomatoes over top for a taste and color boost.

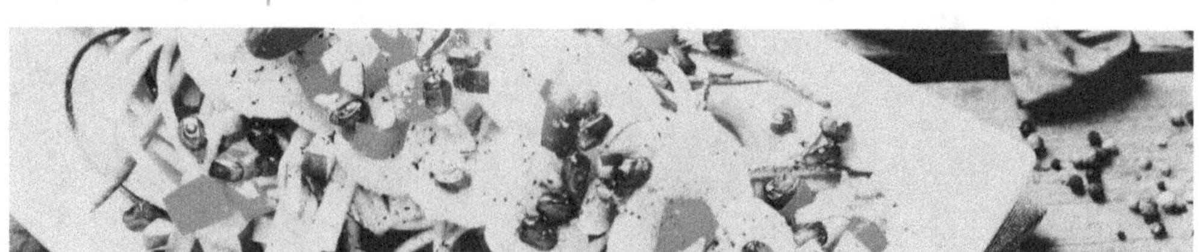

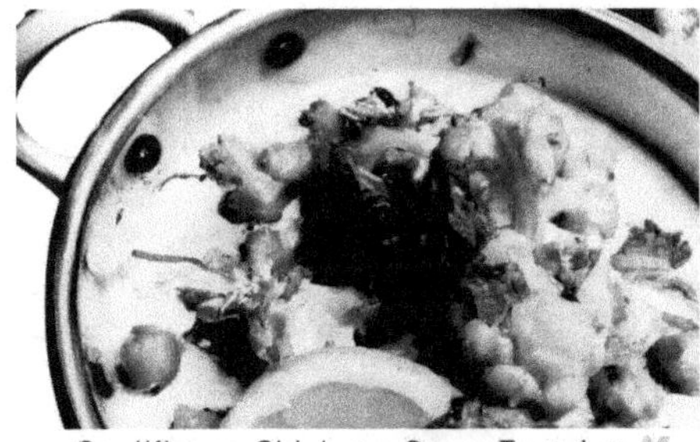

Cauliflower Chickpea Curry. Tasty!

Creamy Cauliflower & Chickpea Curry

Prep ⏰	Cook ⏰	Serves
15 minutes	25 minutes	4

Embark on a culinary adventure with my Cauliflower and Chickpea Curry – a delectable PCOS-friendly creation designed to infuse flavor into your nourishment routine. Packed with goodness and a symphony of aromatic spices, this dish is my go-to for a wholesome and satisfying meal.

INGREDIENTS:

- 1 can (15 oz) of chickpeas, drained and rinsed
- 1 finely chopped onion
- 2 minced cloves of garlic
- 1-inch piece of grated fresh ginger
- 1 can (15 oz) of diced tomatoes
- 1 cup of washed and chopped spinach leaves
- 1 tablespoon of olive oil
- 1 teaspoon of ground turmeric
- 1 teaspoon of ground cumin
- 1 teaspoon of ground coriander
- 1/2 teaspoon of chili powder (adjust to taste)
- Salt and pepper to taste
- Fresh cilantro leaves for garnish

Curry promises to bring both delight and health-conscious goodness to your table.

INSTRUCTIONS

1. Sauté the Aromatics: Start by heating olive oil in a pan. Sauté the finely chopped onion until translucent, then add minced garlic and grated ginger for another fragrant layer.

2. Spice It Up: Mix in ground turmeric, cumin, coriander, and chili powder. Let the spices mingle for a minute, creating a tantalizing base for your curry.

3. Add Tomatoes and Chickpeas: Introduce diced tomatoes and chickpeas, ensuring an even coat with the aromatic spice mix. Let it simmer for 10-15 minutes, allowing the flavors to meld and the sauce to thicken.

4. Incorporate Spinach: Gently fold in chopped spinach, letting it become tender in the curry's warmth. Season with salt and pepper as you like.

5. Garnish and Serve: Your Chickpea and Spinach Curry is ready! Serve it hot, garnished with fresh cilantro leaves for an extra burst of flavor.

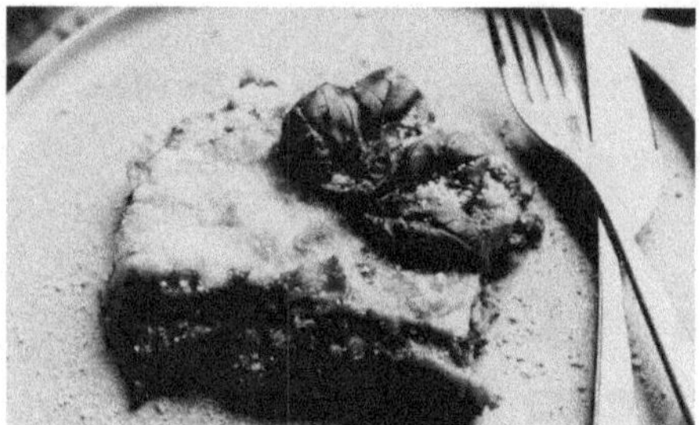

Eggplant Lasagna: Layers of delight.

Prep ⏰
30 minutes

Cook ⏰
30 minutes

Serves
4-6

Eggplant Lasagna

Ah, my Eggplant Lasagna, a traditional favorite made PCOS-friendly. Get ready for a delicious trip that supports your wellness objectives!

INGREDIENTS:

- 2 large eggplants, sliced lengthwise
- 1 pound ground turkey (or lean ground meat of your choice)
- 1 onion, finely chopped
- 3 cloves garlic, minced
- 2 cups tomato sauce (look for low-sugar or homemade options)
- 1 teaspoon dried oregano
- 1 teaspoon dried basil
- Salt and pepper to taste
- 2 cups ricotta cheese
- 1 cup grated mozzarella cheese
- Fresh basil leaves for garnish

Savor the flavorful option that is PCOS-friendly without sacrificing flavor—my eggplant lasagna. For a well-rounded dinner, try serving it with a light cucumber salad or a side of mixed greens. Cheers to enjoying every meal without any guilt!

INSTRUCTIONS

1. Prepare Eggplant Slices: Lay out the eggplant slices on a paper towel and sprinkle with salt. Let them sit for about 15 minutes to draw out excess moisture. Pat them dry.
2. Brown Ground Turkey: In a skillet, brown the ground turkey over medium heat. Add chopped onions and minced garlic, cooking until the onions are translucent.
3. Layering: In a baking dish, start with a layer of eggplant slices, followed by a layer of ground turkey mixture, ricotta cheese, and tomato sauce. Repeat until you've used all your ingredients, finishing with a layer of tomato sauce on top. Sprinkle mozzarella cheese over the final layer.
4. Bake: Bake in a preheated oven at 375°F (190°C) for 25-30 minutes or until the cheese is bubbly and golden.
5. Serve: Garnish with fresh basil leaves and let it cool for a few minutes before serving.

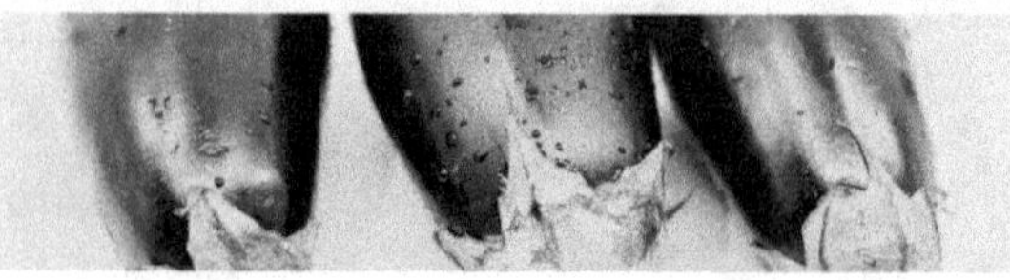

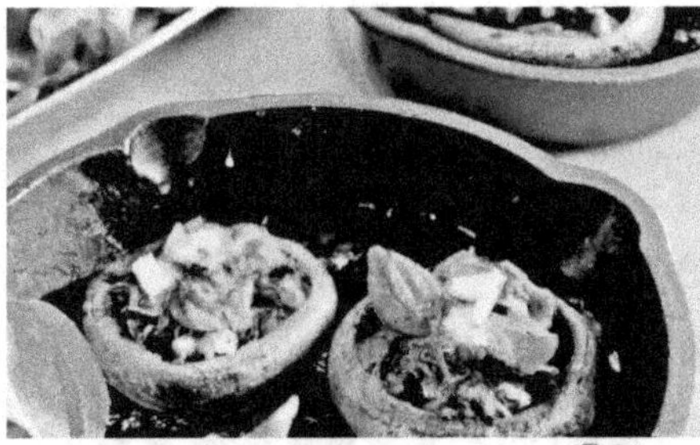

Spinach Feta Portobellos. Yum!

Prep ⏰	**Cook** ⏰	**Serves**
15 minutes	20 minutes	2-4

Spinach & Feta Stuffed Portobello Mushrooms

Hi there! Come along for a taste adventure with my PCOS-friendly and incredibly delicious Spinach & Feta Stuffed Portobello Mushrooms.

INGREDIENTS:

- 4 large Portobello mushrooms with their stems removed
- 2 cups chopped fresh spinach
- 1 cup of crumbled feta cheese
- 1/2 cup of diced cherry tomatoes
- 2 minced garlic cloves
- 1 teaspoon of dried oregano
- 2 tablespoons of olive oil
- Season with salt and pepper
- Garnish with fresh basil leaves

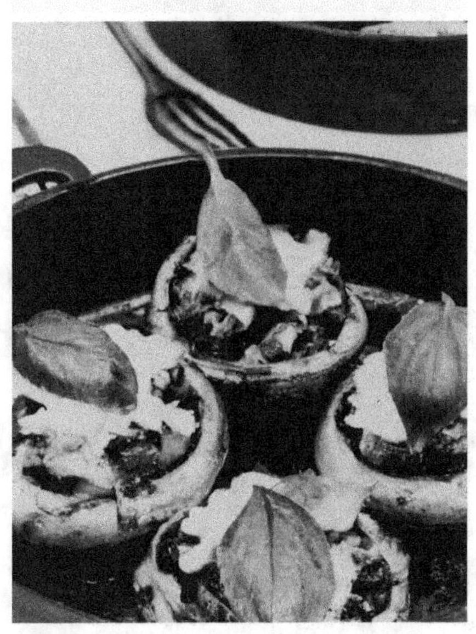

INSTRUCTIONS

1. Get the portobellos ready: Turn the oven on to 375°F, or 190°C. After cleaning, cut off the stems from the Portobello mushrooms.
2. Put the Filling in a Saute: Minced garlic should be sautéed in olive oil in a skillet over medium heat until fragrant. Cook the spinach until it wilts by adding the diced tomatoes and chopped spinach. Add oregano, salt, and pepper for seasoning.
3. Pack the Mushrooms: Arrange the caps of Portobello on a baking sheet. Spoon a good amount of the sautéed spinach mixture into each cap. Add crumbled feta on top.
4. Bake: Bake for 15 to 20 minutes, or until the cheese is brown and the mushrooms are soft, in a preheated oven.
5. Serve: Before serving, garnish with fresh basil leaves.

Here it is: my savory, flavor-bursting Portobello Mushrooms stuffed with spinach and feta. They are also PCOS-friendly. Serve them as an appetizer or as a side dish with quinoa salad. Salutations!

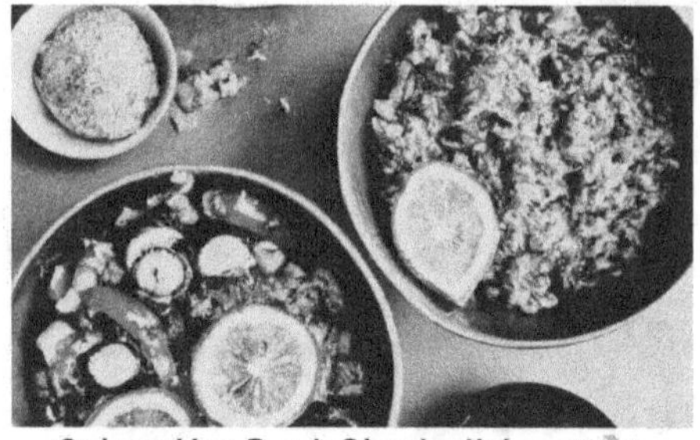

Quinoa Veg Bowl: Simply divine. 🍲🌱

Prep ⏰	Cook ⏰	Serves
15 minutes	25 minutes	2

Quinoa & Roasted Vegetable Buddha Bowl

Greetings, kitchen comrades! Today, let's whip up a Quinoa & Roasted Vegetable Buddha Bowl – a PCOS-friendly feast that's both nourishing and oh-so-satisfying.

INGREDIENTS:

- 1 cup quinoa, rinsed
- 2 cups broccoli florets
- 1 bell pepper, sliced
- 1 zucchini, sliced
- 1 carrot, julienned
- 2 tablespoons olive oil
- 1 teaspoon cumin
- 1 teaspoon paprika
- Salt and pepper to taste
- 1/2 cup hummus
- Fresh lemon wedges for serving

INSTRUCTIONS

1. Preheat & Cook Quinoa: Rinse quinoa under cold water. Cook according to package instructions.
2. Roast the Veggies: Preheat your oven to 425°F (220°C). Toss broccoli, bell pepper, zucchini, and carrot with olive oil, cumin, paprika, salt, and pepper. Roast for 20-25 minutes until veggies are tender and slightly charred.
3. Assemble the Bowl: In serving bowls, layer quinoa and top with the roasted veggies. Add a dollop of hummus in the center.
4. Serve: Drizzle with extra olive oil, sprinkle with salt and pepper, and serve with a wedge of fresh lemon.

There you have it – my Quinoa & Roasted Vegetable Buddha Bowl! It's a PCOS-friendly powerhouse filled with protein, fiber, and a burst of flavors. Customize it with your favorite veggies and savor the goodness. Enjoy this bowlful of delight! 🌱🍲

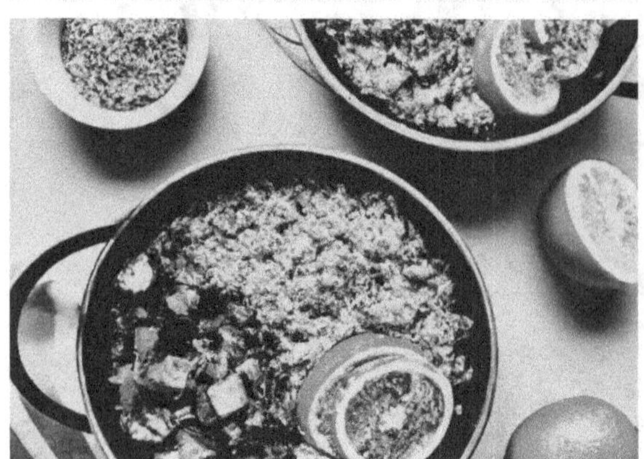

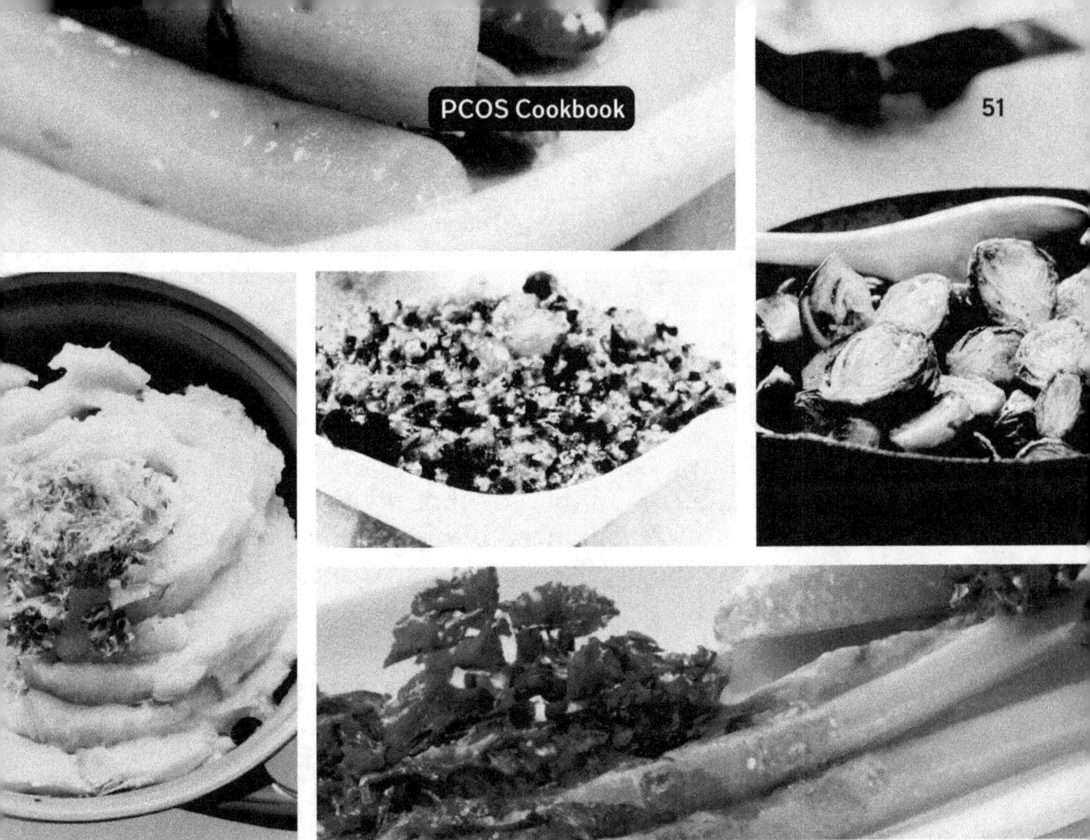

Side Dish Wonders: A symphony of flavors.

8

SATISFYING SIDES

Looking for satisfying and PCOS-friendly side dishes to add flair to your meals? Enjoy these delicious dishes: Balsamic Glazed Carrots, Lemon Herb Asparagus, Mashed Sweet Potatoes, Quinoa and Black Bean Pilaf, and Garlic Roasted Brussels Sprouts. Your dining experience will be both fun and health-conscious thanks to these delectable sides that perfectly balance your main entrees. Together, let's set off on a voyage of delectable and nutritious options!

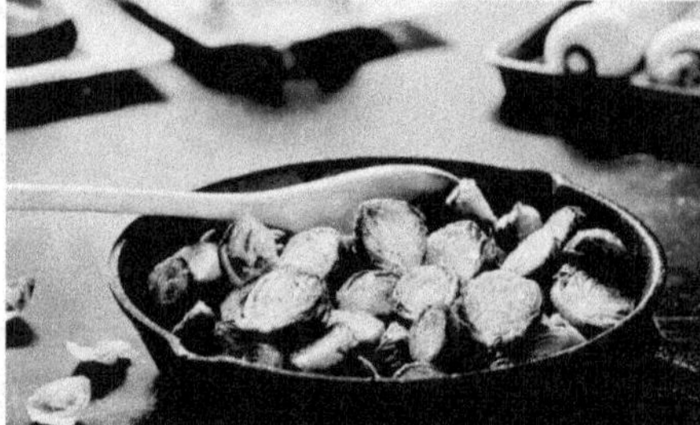

Garlic Roasted Brussels: Flavorful bites.

Prep ⏱	**Cook** ⏱	**Serves**
10 minutes	20-25 minutes	4

Garlic Roasted Brussels Sprouts

Take a taste trip with my Garlic Roasted Brussels Sprouts, a tasty and nutritious side dish that is suitable for those with PCOS. The natural flavors of these sprouts are enhanced by their exquisite oven roasting. This recipe, which is full of vital nutrients, is a healthy addition to your PCOS-conscious lifestyle as well as a culinary treat.

INGREDIENTS:

- 1 pound of chopped and halved brussels sprouts
- 2 tablespoons of olive oil
- 3 minced garlic cloves
- Salt and pepper to taste
- Optional: grated parmesan cheese for garnish

INSTRUCTIONS

1. Set the oven temperature to 400°F, or 200°C.
2. In a bowl toss the Brussels sprouts in a bowl with olive oil, chopped garlic, salt, and pepper until evelyn coated
3. Arrange the sprouts on a baking sheet in a single layer.
4. Roast for 20 to 25 minutes, stirring halfway through to ensure equal cooking, or until they are golden brown and crispy around the edges.
5. Before serving, if desired, top with grated Parmesan cheese.

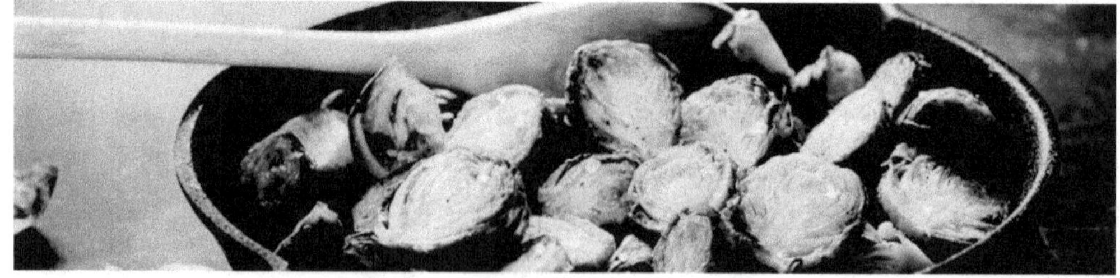

For a filling and well-balanced dinner, try these Garlic Roasted Brussels Sprouts with your favorite lean protein, such as salmon or grilled chicken. This easy-to-make but delicious side dish will brighten up your meal and add a healthy dose of flavor. Have fun! 🌿

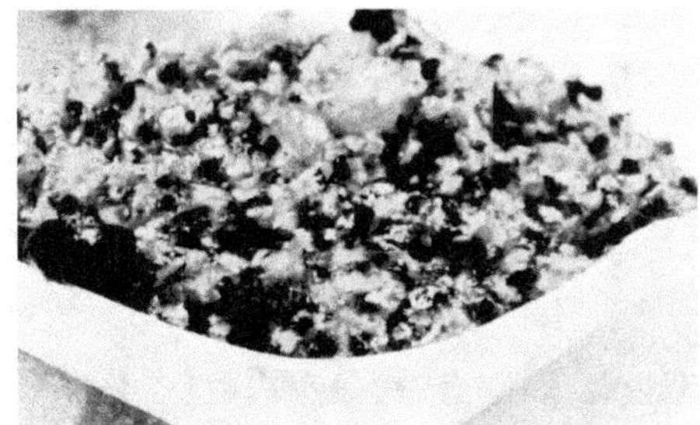

Prep ⏰
10 minutes

Cook ⏰
20 minutes

Serves
4

Quinoa and Black Bean Pilaf

Nutrient-packed perfection.

Up your side dish game with this Quinoa and Black Bean Pilaf, a healthy and PCOS-friendly choice that combines the protein-richness of black beans with the deliciousness of quinoa. Not only is this aromatic pilaf a delicious side dish for your meals, but it's also a healthy option for people with PCOS. Now let's go to work making this easy but filling dinner.

INGREDIENTS:

- 1 cup of rinsed quinoa
- 2 cups of vegetable broth
- 1 can (15 oz.) of drained and washed black beans
- 1 cup of frozen or fresh corn kernels
- 1 chopped red bell pepper
- 1 teaspoon ground cumin
- 1 teaspoon chili powder
- Season with salt and pepper
- Garnish with fresh cilantro, if desired

INSTRUCTIONS

1. Combine the vegetable broth and quinoa in a medium-sized saucepan. After bringing to a boil, lower the heat, cover, and simmer the quinoa for 15 minutes, or until it is tender and the liquid has been absorbed.
2. Sauté the diced red bell pepper, corn, and black beans in another pan until they are thoroughly heated.
3. Include the cooked quinoa in the mixture of vegetables and beans.
4. Add chili powder, ground cumin, pepper, and salt to the pilaf. Mix thoroughly to blend.
5. If preferred, garnish with fresh cilantro.

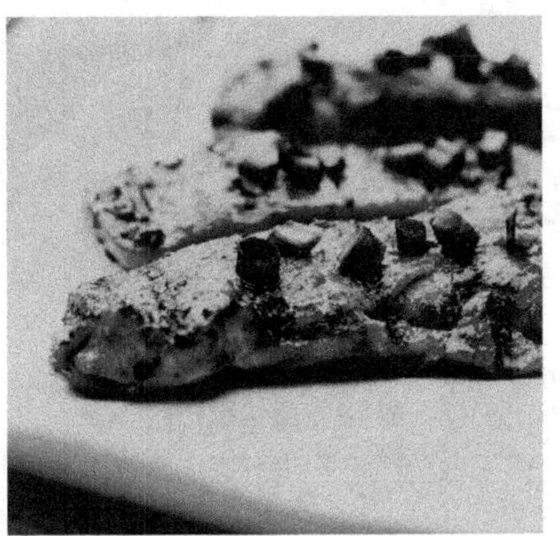

Suggestion: For a filling and high-protein supper, try this Quinoa and Black Bean Pilaf with some grilled chicken or avocado on the side. This PCOS-friendly side improves your general health in addition to adding diversity to your meal. Savor each bite's explosion of flavors and nutrients!

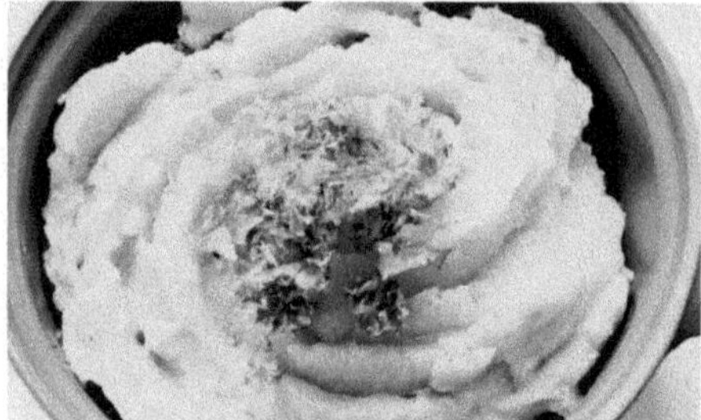

Sweet Potato Mash. Pure comfort. 🥄😊

Prep ⏰	Cook ⏰	Serves
15 minutes	15 minutes	4

Mashed Sweet Potatoes

Welcome to a comforting classic with a nutritious twist—my Mashed Sweet Potatoes! Packed with PCOS-friendly benefits and a touch of natural sweetness, these mashed sweet potatoes are sure to become a staple in your satisfying sides repertoire. Let's dive into creating this velvety, flavorful dish that not only supports your well-being but also adds a delightful touch to your meals.

INGREDIENTS:

- 4 medium-sized sweet potatoes, peeled and cubed
- 2 tablespoons unsalted butter or coconut oil
- 1/4 cup almond milk or any preferred milk
- 1 tablespoon pure maple syrup (optional)
- Salt and cinnamon to taste
- Chopped fresh parsley for garnish (optional)

INSTRUCTIONS

1. Boil or steam the sweet potato cubes until fork-tender.
2. Drain the sweet potatoes and transfer them to a mixing bowl.
3. Add butter or coconut oil, almond milk, and pure maple syrup (if using).
4. Mash the sweet potatoes until smooth and creamy.
5. Season with salt and a pinch of cinnamon, adjusting to your taste preference.
6. Garnish with chopped fresh parsley if desired.

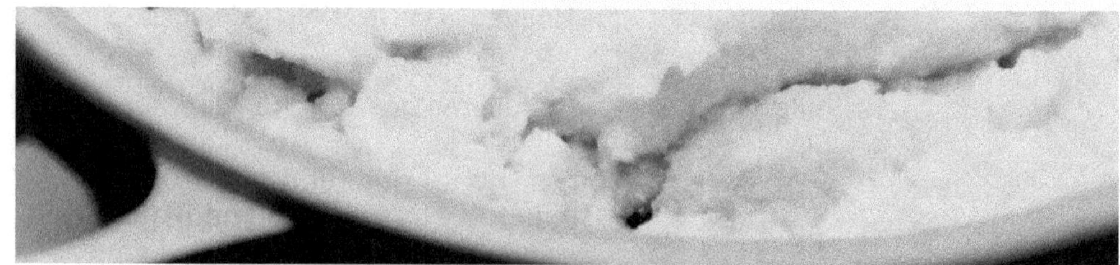

These Mashed Sweet Potatoes pair wonderfully with grilled chicken or roasted vegetables, adding a wholesome touch to your PCOS-friendly meals. Embrace the heartiness and flavor of this side dish that not only satisfies your taste buds but also supports your overall well-being. Enjoy this comforting classic with a healthy twist! 🥄

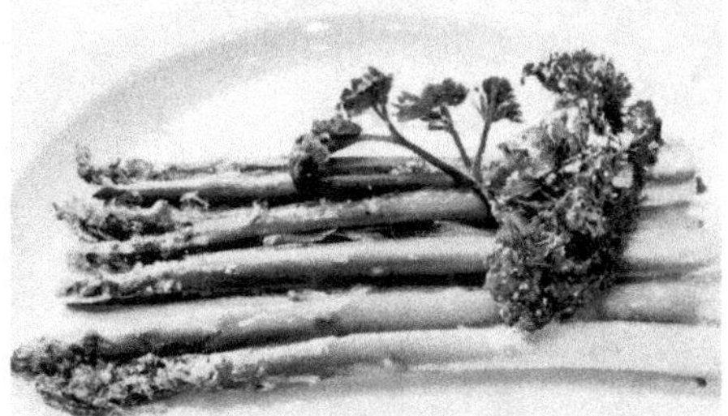

L.H. Asparagus. Zesty goodness.

Prep ⏰ 10 minutes   **Cook** ⏰ 15 minutes   **Serves** 4

Lemon Herb Asparagus

Let's brighten up your plate with a burst of freshness—my Lemon Herb Asparagus! This PCOS-friendly side dish not only brings vibrant flavors to your table but also supports your well-being with nutritious goodness. Get ready to elevate your meals with this simple and delightful recipe.

INGREDIENTS:

- 1 bunch of fresh asparagus, tough ends trimmed
- 2 tablespoons olive oil
- Zest of 1 lemon
- 2 tablespoons fresh lemon juice
- 2 cloves garlic, minced
- 1 teaspoon dried thyme
- Salt and black pepper to taste
- Fresh parsley for garnish (optional)

INSTRUCTIONS

1. Preheat your oven to 400°F (200°C).
2. Place asparagus on a baking sheet, drizzle with olive oil, and toss to coat evenly.
3. Sprinkle lemon zest, lemon juice, minced garlic, dried thyme, salt, and pepper over the asparagus, ensuring an even distribution of flavors.
4. Roast in the preheated oven for 12-15 minutes, or until the asparagus is tender yet still crisp.
5. Garnish with fresh parsley if desired.

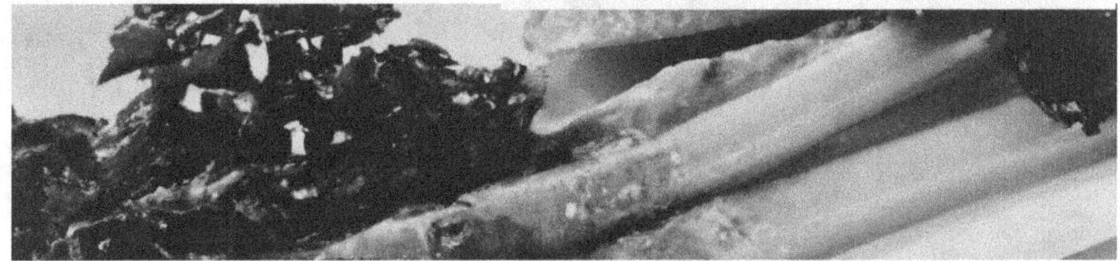

This Lemon Herb Asparagus pairs wonderfully with grilled fish or a lean protein of your choice, making it a versatile and refreshing addition to your PCOS-friendly meals. Embrace the delightful combination of citrusy zest and savory herbs, adding a nutritious touch to your plate. Enjoy this vibrant side dish that not only delights your taste buds but also contributes to your overall well-being!

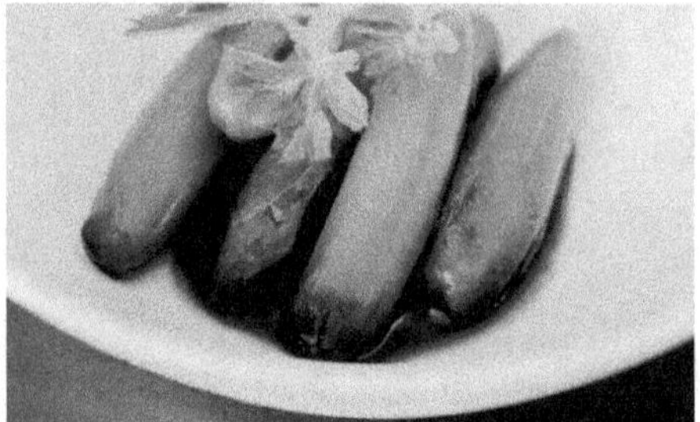

Balsamic Glazed Carrots. Sweet delight!

Prep ⏲
10 minutes

Cook ⏲
20-25 minutes

Serves
4

Balsamic Glazed Carrots

A taste explosion is waiting for you when you say goodbye to boring carrots and hello to the tantalizing blend of balsamic glaze. These glazed carrots are a great option for a side dish that fits with PCOS-friendly eating because they give a hint of sweetness to your meal.

INGREDIENTS:

- 1 pound of washed and peeled baby carrots
- 2 tablespoons of balsamic vinegar
- 1 tablespoon of olive oil
- 1 tablespoon of honey
- Salt and black pepper To taste
- (Optional) fresh parsley for garnish

INSTRUCTIONS

1. Set the oven temperature to 400°F, or 200°C.
2. Combine the olive oil, honey, balsamic vinegar, salt, and pepper in a bowl.
3. Toss the baby carrots in the balsamic mixture until they are evenly coated
4. Spread the carrots out in a single layer on a baking pan.
5. Roast, stirring halfway through, in the preheated oven for 20 to 25 minutes, or until the carrots are soft.
6. If preferred, garnish with fresh parsley.

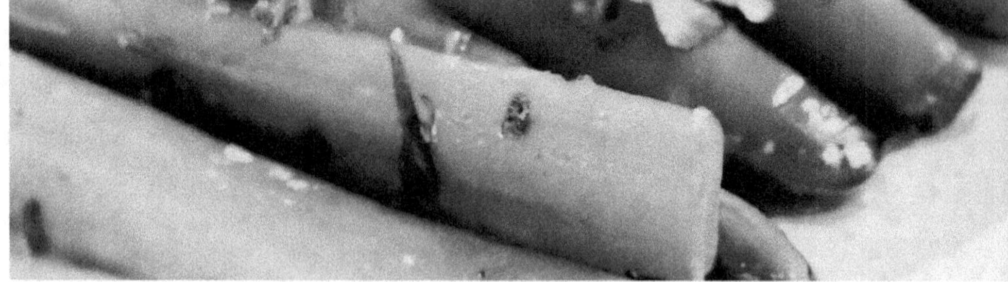

Suggestions: These Carrots with Balsamic Glaze are a delicious side dish for grilled fish or roasted chicken. Their flavor profile, which combines sweetness and tanginess, gives your dish a distinctive twist and supports a PCOS-friendly lifestyle. Taste and nutrients come together at your table with these glazed carrots! Lift your plate with this easy but tasty side!

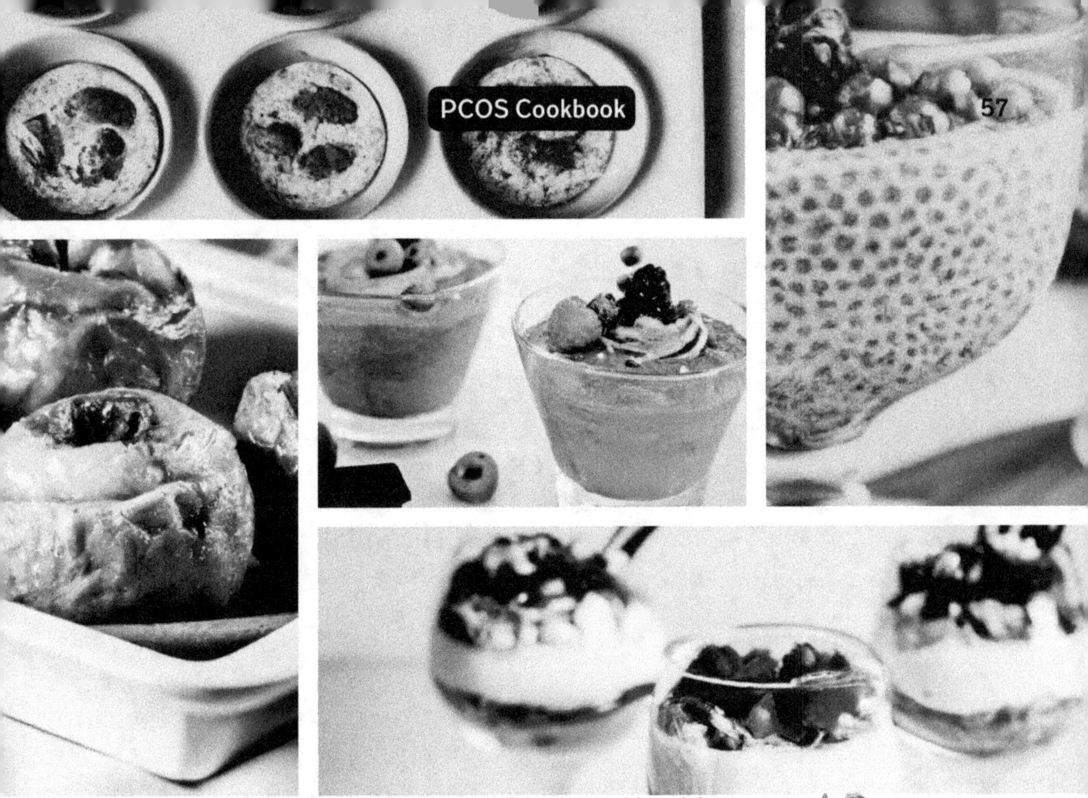

PCOS-Friendly Desserts: Sweet and healthy treats. 🍰🍓

9

HEALTHY DESSERTS

Enjoy sugar without feeling guilty with my Healthy Desserts, a selection designed for people managing PCOS. These delicacies are made to fulfill your sweet need while adhering to PCOS-friendly options. They range from the velvety Dark Chocolate Avocado Mousse to the refreshing Chia Seed Pudding with Berries. Feel the warmth of a Cinnamon Baked Apple, sink into a delicious Coconut and Berry Parfait, and savor the deliciousness of Almond Butter Banana Bites.

Adopting a health-conscious lifestyle is a genuinely pleasurable experience thanks to these treats. Let us relish each morsel while promoting our overall health! 🍏🍎

Prep ⏰
5 minutes

Cook ⏰
0 minutes

Serves
2

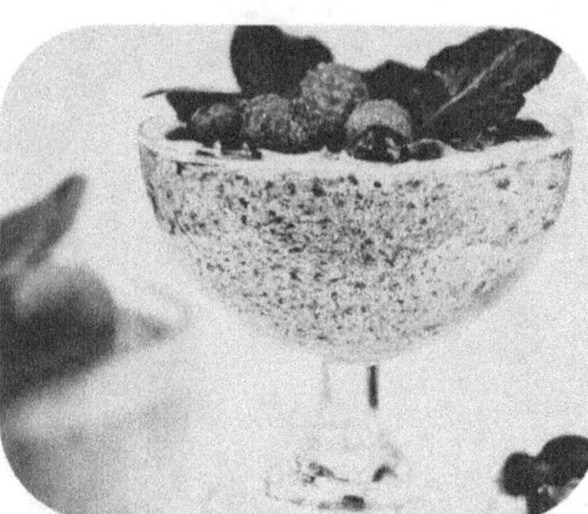

Chia Berry Pudding: Simply divine. 🍓

Chia Seed Pudding with Berries

Take a pleasantly healthy journey with my Chia Seed Pudding with Berries, a PCOS-friendly delicacy that blends delectable flavors and nourishing richness. The small chia seeds thicken into a pudding-like consistency, giving a wonderful texture that complements the sweetness of fresh berries. This dish, which is high in omega-3 fatty acids and fiber, is not only delicious but also good for your health.

INGREDIENTS:

- 1/4 cup chia seeds
- 1 cup unsweetened almond milk
- 1 tablespoon honey or maple syrup (optional).
- 1/2 teaspoon vanilla extract
- A handful of fresh berries (strawberries, blueberries, raspberries)

INSTRUCTIONS

1. In a mixing bowl, combine chia seeds, almond milk, honey or maple syrup (if using), and vanilla extract.
2. Give it a good stir and let it settle for a few minutes.
3. Stir again after 10 minutes to avoid clumping, then cover and chill for at least 2-3 hours, or overnight.
4. Before serving, give it a final swirl. Decorate with fresh berries.

Indulge in this guilt-free pleasure that is both delicious and nutritionally dense. Serve as a refreshing dessert after dinner or a delicious brunch alternative. The adaptable Chia Seed Pudding with Berries is an excellent canvas for your imagination—try adding nuts or a drizzle of nut butter for an extra layer of taste and texture. Enjoy the healthy goodness and relish every bite! 🌱🍓

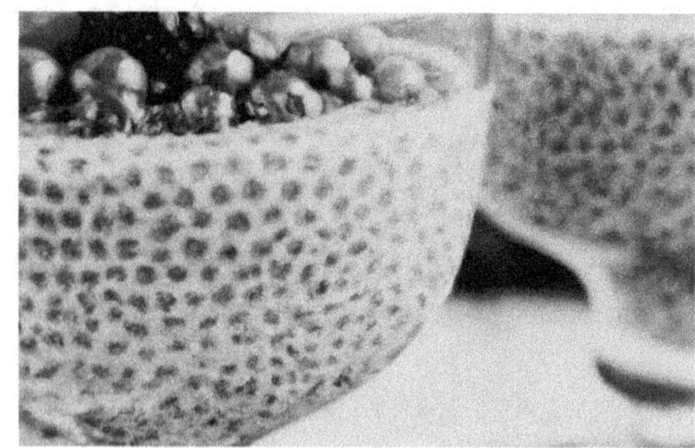

Prep ⏰	**Cook** ⏰	**Serves**
10 minutes	0 minutes	4

Dark Chocolate Avocado Mousse

Embark on a pleasant indulgent journey with my PCOS-friendly Dark Chocolate Avocado Mousse —a guilt-free dessert that flawlessly marries rich chocolatey pleasure with the nutritious benefits of avocados. This velvety delicacy not only satisfies your sweet craving but also feeds your body. Avocado gives a creamy texture, while dark chocolate offers a delicious flavor, resulting in a beautiful mix of indulgence and health.

INGREDIENTS:

- 2 ripe avocados
- 1/4 cup cocoa powder (unsweetened)
- 1/4 cup melted dark chocolate chips
- 1/4 cup maple syrup or honey
- 1 teaspoon vanilla extract
- A pinch of salt
- Optional garnish: fresh berries

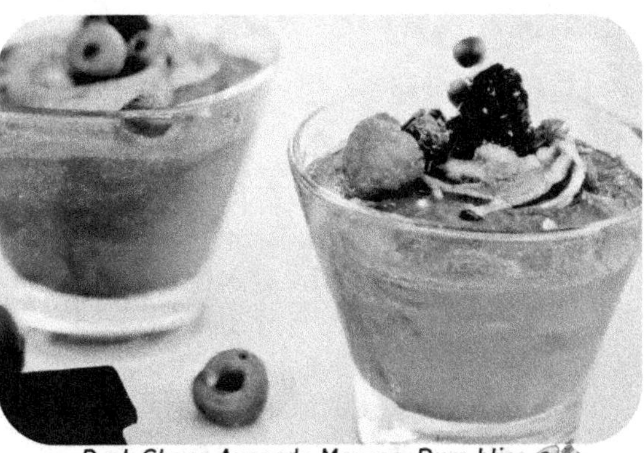

Dark Choco Avocado Mousse. Pure bliss.

INSTRUCTIONS

1. In a blender or food processor, add ripe avocados, cocoa powder, dark chocolate melted, maple syrup or honey, vanilla essence, and a touch of salt.
2. Mix until smooth and creamy, scraping down the sides as needed.
3. Check the sweetness and adjust it if necessary.
4. Spoon the mousse into serving glasses and chill for at least 1-2 hours.
5. If preferred, garnish with fresh berries prior to serving.

Each spoonful of this Dark Chocolate Avocado Mousse contains a wonderful mix of velvety chocolate and creamy avocado. This dish is both delicious and healthy, making it ideal for satisfying your sweet cravings. Serve it as an elegant dessert or as a special treat. A sprinkling of nuts or a dollop of coconut whipped cream will add a touch of elegance. Enjoy guilt-free enjoyment!

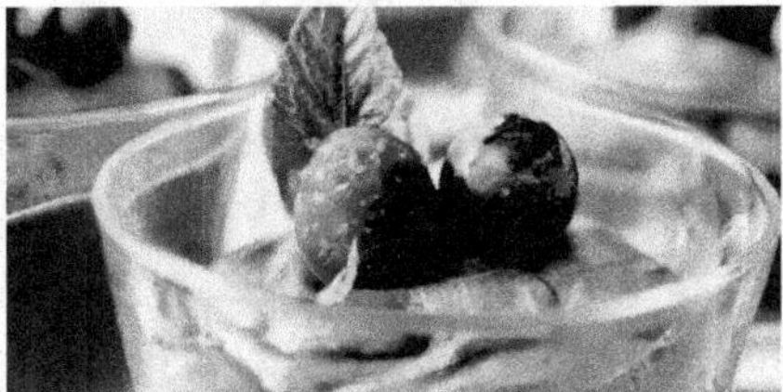

Prep ⏰	**Cook** ⏰	**Serves**
10 minutes	24-30 minutes	4

Baked Apple with Cinnamon

Enjoy the comforting aroma of my PCOS-friendly Baked Apple with Cinnamon, a nourishing dish that combines the natural sweetness of apples with the warmth of cinnamon. This simple but delectable treat provides a sense of comfort and sustenance to your taste, making it the ideal guilt-free indulgence.

INGREDIENTS:

- 4 medium-sized apples (like Gala or Honeycrisp)
- 2 tablespoons melted butter or coconut oil.
- 2 teaspoons of ground cinnamon
- 2 tablespoons of chopped nuts (walnuts, almonds, or pecans).
- 2 tablespoons dried cranberries or raisins (optional)
- Optional: sprinkle with honey or maple syrup.

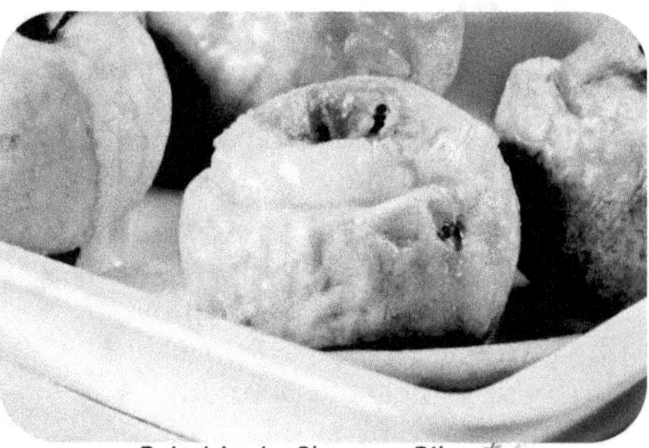

Baked Apple, Cinnamon Bliss. 🍎✨

INSTRUCTIONS

1. Preheat the oven to 375° F (190° C).
2. Core the apples and arrange in a baking dish.
3. In a small mixing dish, combine melted coconut oil or butter and ground cinnamon.
4. Brush the cinnamon mixture over each apple, ensuring that it is thoroughly coated.
5. Sprinkle the apples with the chopped nuts and raisins (if using).
6. Bake for 25 to 30 minutes, or until the apples are soft.
7. Take out of the oven, pour with honey or maple syrup, and serve warm.

Enjoy the heartwarming sweetness of Baked Apple with Cinnamon, a sweet and satisfying dessert that captures the essence of autumn. This PCOS-friendly dessert is not only simple to prepare, but it also allows you to enjoy the nutritious flavors of nature. Serve it as is or with a dollop of Greek yogurt for extra richness. Feel free to indulge in warm cinnamon-kissed apples! 🍎✨

Prep ⏰
10 minutes

Cook ⏰
0 minutes

Serves
2

Coconut & Berries Parfait

Let me show you how I make a delicious PCOS-friendly treat: Coconut and Berry Parfait. This decadent dessert combines the richness of coconut with the burst of flavors from fresh berries, resulting in a symphony for your taste buds. Let's explore the realm of guilt-free indulgence that not only fulfills your sweet desires but also supports your PCOS management goals.

INGREDIENTS:

- 1 cup coconut yogurt (dairy-free for a vegan alternative)
- One cup of mixed berries (strawberries, blueberries, raspberries)
- 2 tablespoons shredded, unsweetened coconut
- 2 tablespoons of chopped nuts (almonds, pistachios, or your preference)
- A sprinkle of honey or maple syrup is optional.

Coconut Berry Parfait: A treat! 🥥🍓

INSTRUCTIONS

1. In serving glasses or jars, begin by layering a teaspoon of coconut yogurt.
2. Add a layer of mixed berries, making sure they are well distributed.
3. Add shredded coconut and chopped nuts on top.
4. Continue adding layers until the glass is full, then top with berries and nuts.
5. For extra sweetness, drizzle with honey or maple syrup.
6. Refrigerate for at least 30 minutes prior to serving.

Indulge in the velvety sweetness of Coconut and Berry Parfait, a dessert that perfectly balances the richness of coconut with the freshness of berries. This PCOS-friendly pleasure not only treats your taste buds but also improves your overall health. Serve it as a delicious dessert or guilt-free snack. Celebrate the pleasure of life, one parfait at a time! 🥥🍓✨

Prep ⏰
10 minutes

Cook ⏰
0 minutes

Serves
2

Almond Butter Banana Bites

Step into my kitchen, where I'm excited to share a PCOS-friendly delight: Almond Butter Banana Bites. These bite-sized miracles combine creamy almond butter with the natural sweetness of bananas, creating a guilt-free treat that complements your PCOS control path. Let's go on a basic yet enjoyable culinary excursion!

INGREDIENTS:

- 2 ripe bananas
- 4 tablespoons of unsweetened almond butter
- 2 tablespoons of unsweetened shredded coconut.
- 1 spoonful of chia seeds
- A dash of cinnamon is optional.
- Toothpicks for serving

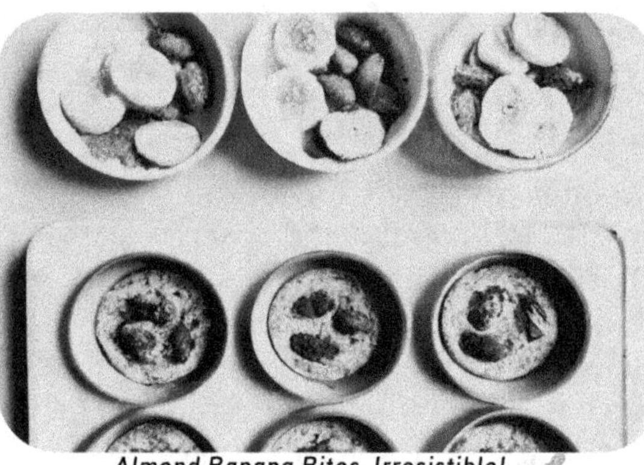

Almond Banana Bites. Irresistible!

INSTRUCTIONS

1. Peel the bananas and slice into bite-sized rounds.
2. Place a thin coating of almond butter on top of each banana round.
3. Top the almond butter with shredded coconut, chia seeds, and (optional) cinnamon.
4. Carefully place toothpicks into each banana bite for convenient serving.
5. Place the bites on a serving tray and chill for at least 15 minutes to allow the flavors to combine.

Enjoy the guilt-free delight of Almond Butter Banana Bites, a PCOS-friendly treat that perfectly combines almond butter's richness with bananas' natural sweetness. These delectable snacks are not only a pleasure for your taste senses, but also a considerate addition to your PCOS-friendly diet. They can be enjoyed as a delicious finale to a meal or as a nutritious snack throughout the day. Dive into the joys of conscious indulgence!

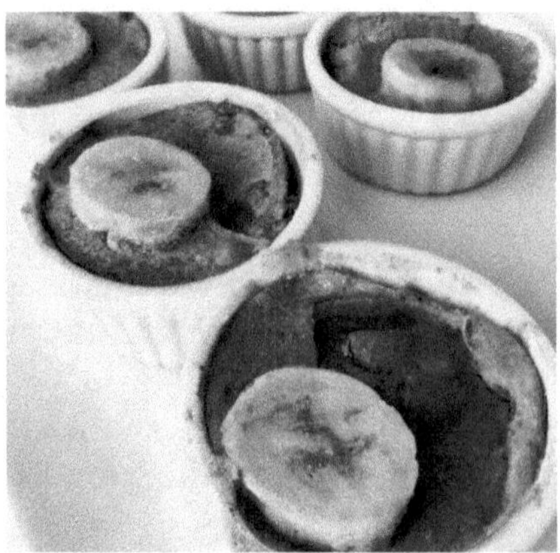

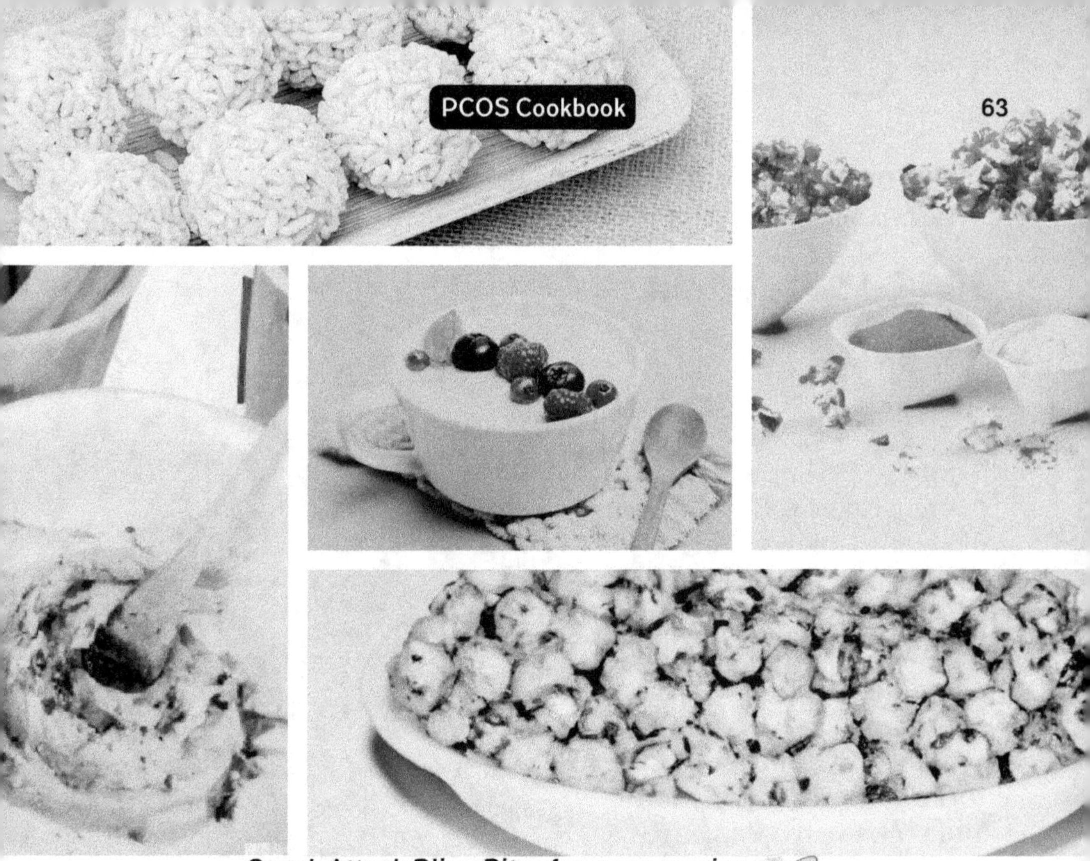

Snack Attack Bliss. Bites for every craving.

10

SNACK ATTACK

Craving a tasty snack without jeopardizing your PCOS-friendly diet? Explore my Snack Attack section for a variety of tasty goodies. From the enticing Almond and Coconut Energy Bites to the savory Edamame Hummus with Veggie Sticks, these snacks are designed with your health in mind. Join me as we explore the ideal combination of flavor and health with options such as Turmeric and Paprika Popcorn, Greek Yogurt and Berry Parfait, and Spicy Roasted Chickpeas. Snacking has never been more delightful and supportive of your PCOS journey.

Prep ⏰	**Cook** ⏰	**Serves**
15 minutes	0 minutes	12 energy bites

Almond & Coconut Energy Bites

Improve your snacking experience with my PCOS-friendly Almond and Coconut Energy Bites! These delicious bites are a nutritious blend of almonds, coconut, and a hint of sweetness, providing the ideal combination of flavor and health benefits. Crafting them is simple, needing little effort and time. In only a few simple steps, you'll have a batch suitable for consumption. This nutritious snack complements your PCOS wellness quest, giving a delicious treat that promotes overall well-being. These energy bites are a great addition to your daily routine, whether shared with friends or enjoyed alone.

INGREDIENTS:

- 1 cup finely chopped almonds
- 1 cup unsweetened shredded coconut.
- 1/3 cup honey or maple syrup.
- Add 1/2 teaspoon vanilla essence and a pinch of salt.

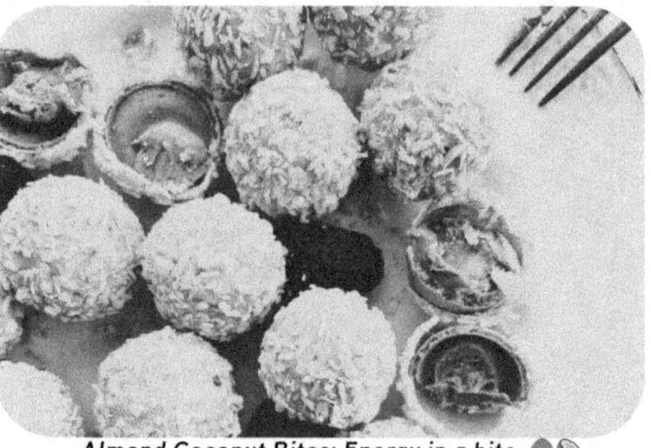

Almond Coconut Bites: Energy in a bite. 🥥🥥

INSTRUCTIONS

1. In a mixing dish, combine the chopped almonds and shredded coconut.
2. Incorporate honey (or maple syrup), vanilla extract, and a bit of salt into the mixture. Stir until thoroughly blended.
3. Using your hands, form the dough into bite-sized balls and set on a lined tray.
4. To set, refrigerate for at least 30 minutes.

Indulge guilt-free in these Almond and Coconut Energy Bites, a delicious snack that not only fills your desires but also promotes PCOS wellness. Enjoy on their own or with a cup of herbal tea for a midday boost! 🌿

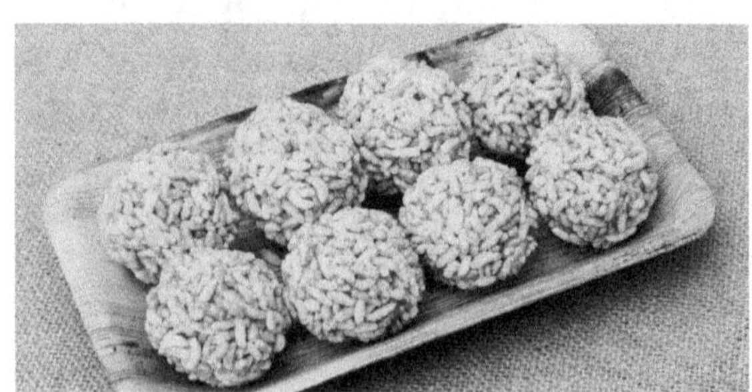

Prep ⏰
10 minutes

Serves
8 energy bites

Edamame Hummus with Veggie Sticks

Enjoy the ideal PCOS-friendly snacking experience with my Edamame Hummus and fresh Veggie Sticks! This delicious hummus, made with protein-rich edamame, adds a pleasant variation to the conventional chickpea-based dip. It's a wonderful alternative for people wishing to meet their nutritional demands while still enjoying a tasty treat. Whether you're fulfilling midday cravings or entertaining visitors, this Edamame Hummus with Veggie Sticks is a healthy option that complements your PCOS wellness goals.

INGREDIENTS:

- 2 cups boiled edamame (shelled)
- 3 tablespoons tahini
- 3 tablespoons olive oil
- 2 cloves chopped garlic
- 1 lemon juice
- 1 teaspoon ground cumin.
- Season to taste with salt and pepper. Dip with carrot sticks, cucumber slices, or bell pepper strips.

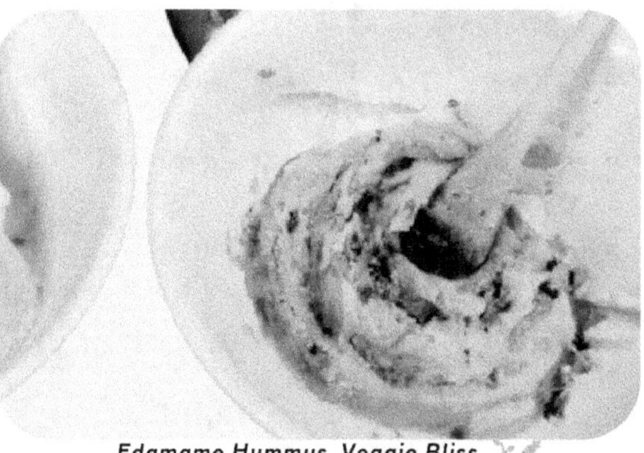

Edamame Hummus, Veggie Bliss.

INSTRUCTIONS

1. In a food processor, mix together the edamame, tahini, olive oil, garlic, lemon juice, ground cumin, salt, and pepper.
2. Blend until smooth, scraping down the sides as needed for a uniform texture.
3. Season to taste and transfer hummus to a serving bowl.
4. Gather a variety of fresh vegetable sticks for dipping.

Enjoy the healthful taste of our Edamame Hummus with Veggie Sticks. It's a protein-packed snack with colorful flavors that can help you live a PCOS-friendly lifestyle. Enjoy this healthy dip with your favorite veggies for a guilt-free delight!

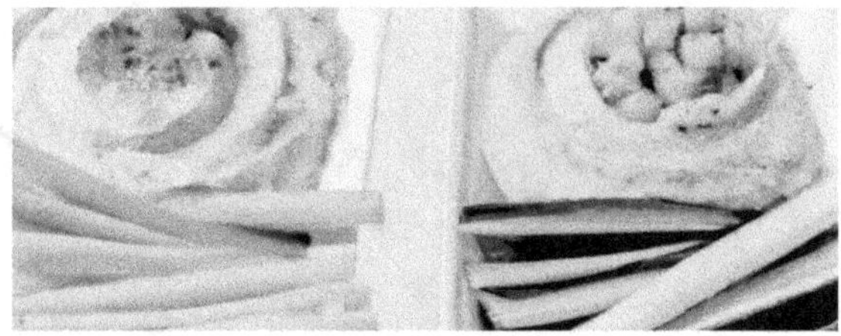

Popcorn with Turmeric & Paprika

Enhance your eating experience with my PCOS-friendly Turmeric and Paprika Popcorn! This delectable popcorn alternative adds a blast of taste and a dose of anti-inflammatory health to your movie night or noon cravings. Turmeric's brilliant color and earthy flavor, mixed with the smokey warmth of paprika, result in a fascinating blend that is not only delicious but also beneficial to your PCOS healing quest. Let us embark on this delectable popcorn experience, assuring the ideal combination of health and taste.

INGREDIENTS:

- 1/2 cup popcorn kernels
- 2 tablespoons coconut oil
- 1 teaspoon ground turmeric.
- 1/2 teaspoon of smoked paprika
- Add salt to taste.

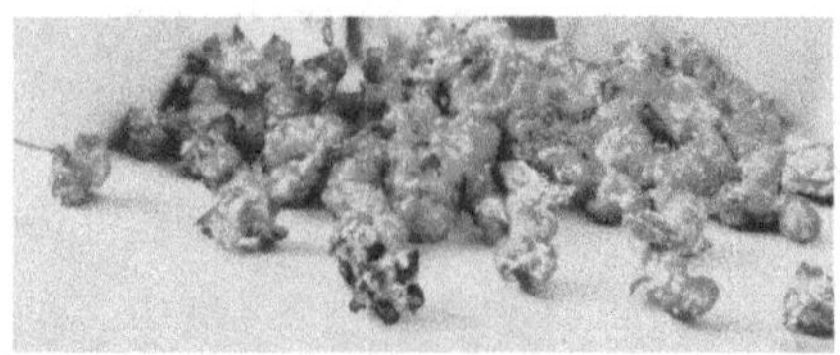

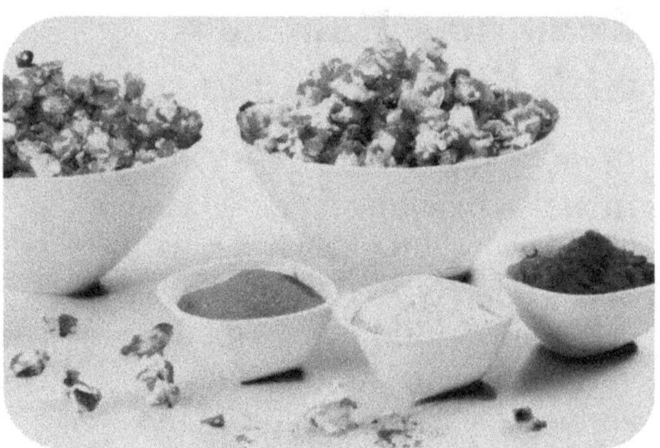

Turmeric Paprika Popcorn. Snack time upgraded! 🍿

INSTRUCTIONS

1. Cook the popcorn kernels in your preferred technique (microwave, stovetop, or air popper).
2. In a small saucepan, heat the coconut oil on low.
3. To make seasoned oil, combine the crushed turmeric and smoked paprika with the heated coconut oil and stir thoroughly.
4. Drizzle the seasoned oil over the popped popcorn and gently toss to coat evenly.
5. Add salt to taste and toss the popcorn once more.

Turmeric & Paprika Popcorn is a guilt-free snack that not only satisfies your desires but also helps you meet your PCOS wellness objectives. Dive into the bright blend of spices and popcorn bliss for a delicious treat that supports a healthy living. Whether it's a nice movie night or a lunchtime snack, this savory popcorn variant will give a healthy twist to your snacking options! 🍿

Prep ⏰
10 minutes

Serves
1

Greek Yogurt and Berry Parfait

Looking for a tasty and healthy snack to help with your PCOS? Let's prepare a Greek Yogurt and Berry Parfait! This parfait mixes the richness of Greek yogurt with the sweetness of berries to create a pleasant treat that is both nutritious and tasty.

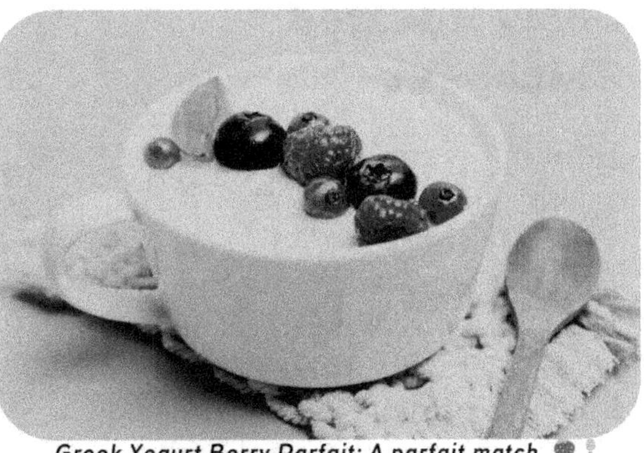

Greek Yogurt Berry Parfait: A parfait match. 🍓

INGREDIENTS:

- 1 cup Greek yogurt.
- 1/2 cup of fresh blueberries
- 1/2 cup of fresh raspberries
- 1/2 cup sliced fresh strawberries.
- 1 tablespoon of honey (optional).
- Granola to top (optional)

INSTRUCTIONS

1. Begin by placing a layer of Greek yogurt on the bottom of a glass or jar.
2. Layer fresh blueberries on top of the yogurt.
3. Finish with a layer of fresh raspberries.
4. Put another layer of yogurt on top of the berries.
5. Garnish the yogurt with cut strawberries.
6. Continue layering until all of the ingredients have been utilized, then finish with a layer of yogurt on top.
7. If preferred, drizzle with honey for an extra sweet finish.
8. For added crunch, top with granola.

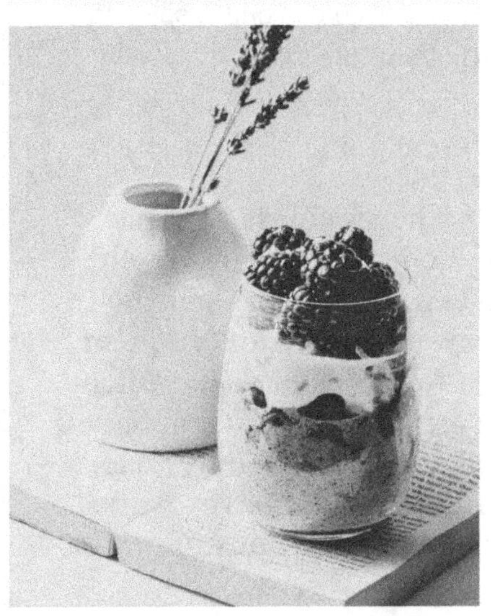

This Greek Yogurt and Berry Parfait is deliciously creamy. It's more than simply a snack; it's a delicious experience that mixes the freshness of berries with the protein boost of Greek yogurt. It can be eaten alone or as a healthy dessert. Let's fuel your health and satisfy your sweet desires in a PCOS-friendly way! 🍓✨

Prep ⏲
10 minutes

Cook ⏲
25-30 minutes

Serves
4

Spicy Roasted Chickpeas

Looking for a crunchy, tasty snack that fits within your PCOS-friendly lifestyle? Enter the world of Spicy Roasted Chickpeas! These roasted chickpeas, which are high in protein and with a spicy taste, are the ideal guilt-free snack to fulfill those cravings.

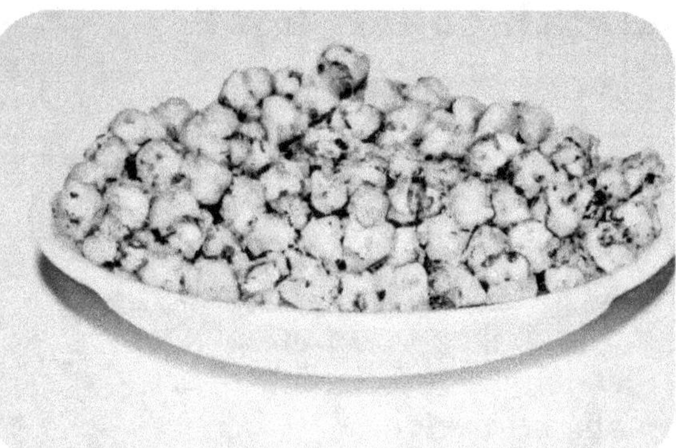
Spicy Roasted Chickpeas: Crunch with a kick. 🌶

INGREDIENTS:

- 2 cans (15 oz) of chickpeas, drained and rinsed
- 2 tablespoons olive oil
- 1 teaspoon cumin
- 1 teaspoon paprika
- 1/2 tsp cayenne pepper (to taste)
- 1/2 teaspoon garlic powder.
- Sprinkle with salt and pepper to taste.

INSTRUCTIONS

1. Heat your oven to 400°F (200°C).
2. Use a paper towel to completely dry the chickpeas.
3. Toss chickpeas with olive oil, cumin, paprika, cayenne pepper, garlic powder, salt, and pepper until equally coated.
4. Spread the chickpeas evenly on a baking sheet.
5. Roast in a preheated oven for 25-30 minutes, or until golden and crispy, stirring the pan halfway through.
6. Remove from the oven and cool before serving.

Enjoy the spiciness of these roasted chickpeas. They're not only a tasty snack on their own, but they also make an excellent addition to salads or as a crunchy topping for soups. This simple and enjoyable PCOS-friendly snack provides flavorful flavor while increasing protein consumption!

🌶

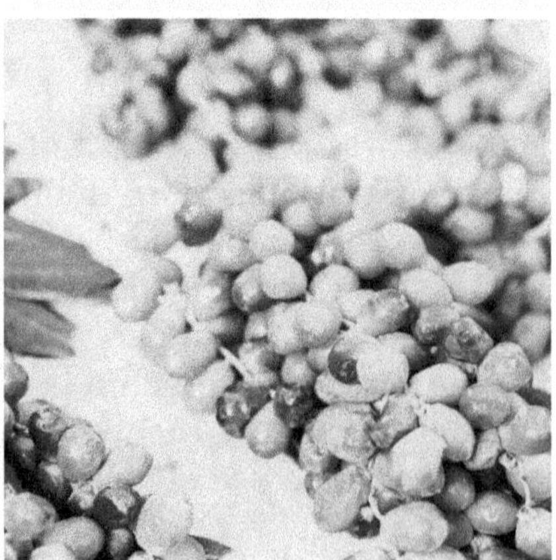

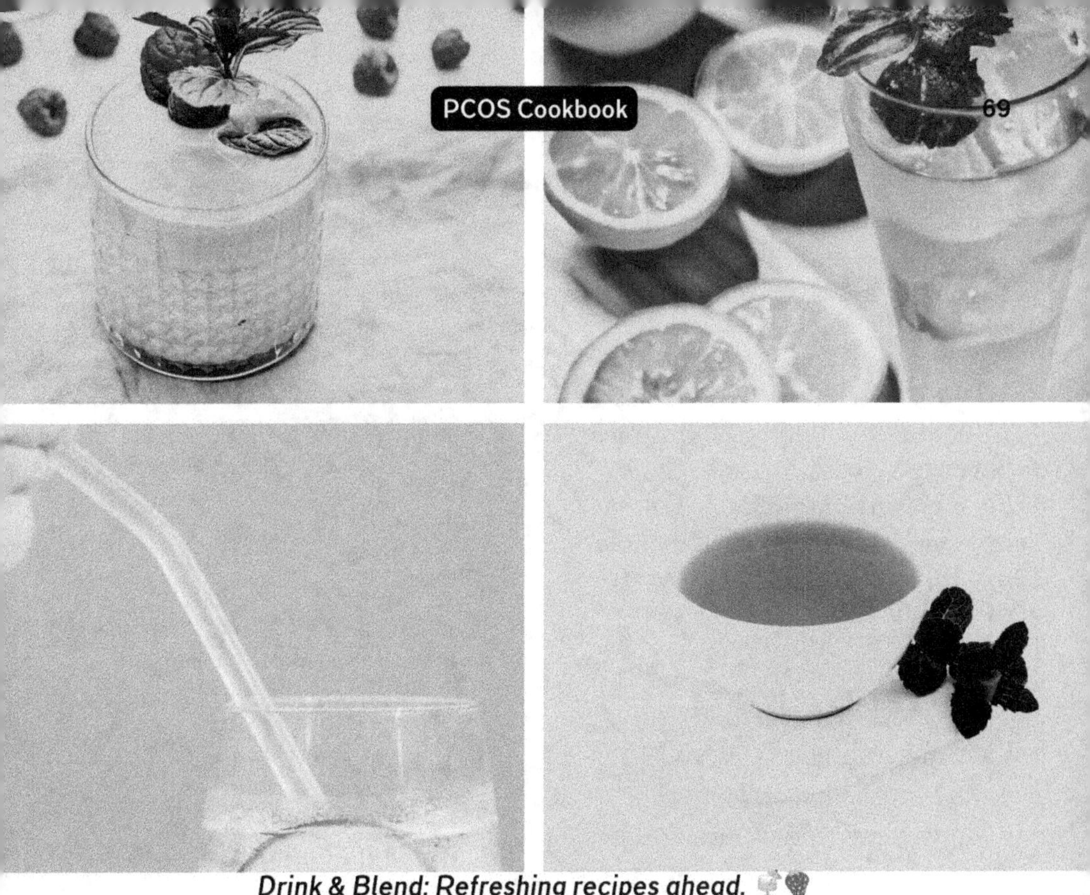

Drink & Blend: Refreshing recipes ahead. 🍹🍓

11

DRINKS & SMOOTHIES

Quench your thirst with bright, PCOS-friendly beverage collection! In this section, I've created delicious drinks to help you stay hydrated while also improving your health. From the antioxidant-rich Green Tea Infusion to the nutrient-dense Berry Blast Smoothie and the purifying Ginger Lemon Detox Water, each sip is intended to be both delightful and helpful. Don't pass up the stimulating Citrus Mint Refresher, which adds zing to your day. Cheers to staying refreshed and nourished with these delicious beverages! 🍵🍓🍐🌿

Prep ⏰
5 minutes

Cook ⏰
5 minutes

Serves
1

Green Tea Infusion

Begin a journey of vigor with my PCOS-friendly Green Tea Infusion. This calming beverage, which is high in antioxidants, not only provides a pleasant pick-me-up but also promotes your overall health.

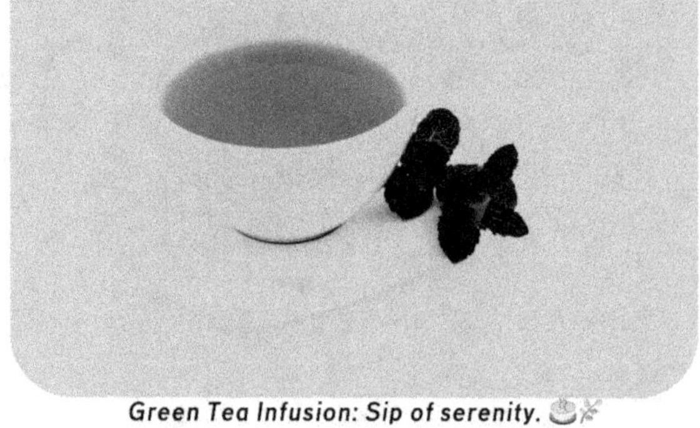

Green Tea Infusion: Sip of serenity. ☕✂

INGREDIENTS:

- 1 green tea bag.
- 1 cup of hot water
- Fresh mint leaves are optional.
- Lemon slices are optional
- Natural sweetener such as honey or stevia (optional)

INSTRUCTIONS

1. Soak the green tea bag in boiling water for 3 to 5 minutes.
2. If preferred, garnish with fresh mint leaves or lemon slices.
3. Optional: sweeten with honey or stevia.
4. Let it cool somewhat before tasting and savoring.

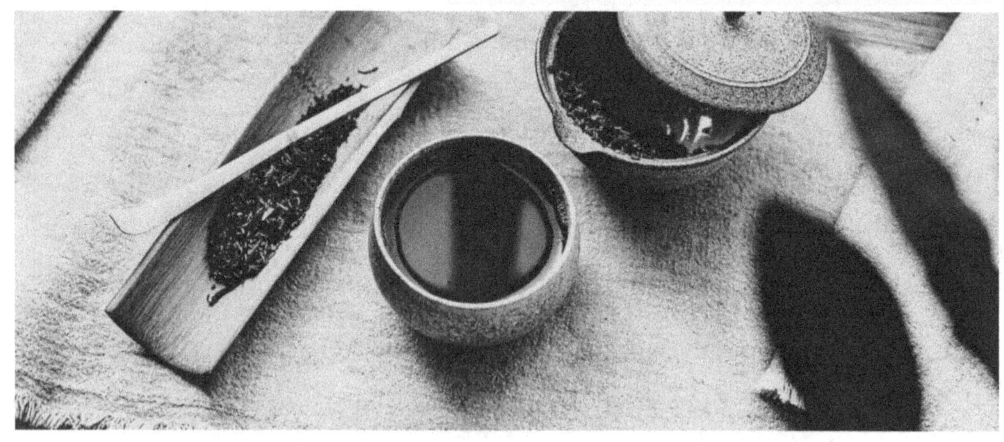

Enjoy this cool Green Tea Infusion as a standalone beverage or with a handful of mixed nuts for a delicious, PCOS-friendly treat. It's a simple practice that provides tranquility and nourishment into your day. ☕✦

Prep ⏰	**Cook** ⏰	**Serves**
5 minutes	0 minutes	1

Berry Blast Smoothie

Enhance your mornings with my PCOS-friendly Berry Blast Smoothie, a vivid blend of tastes and nutrients to get your day started on a healthy note.

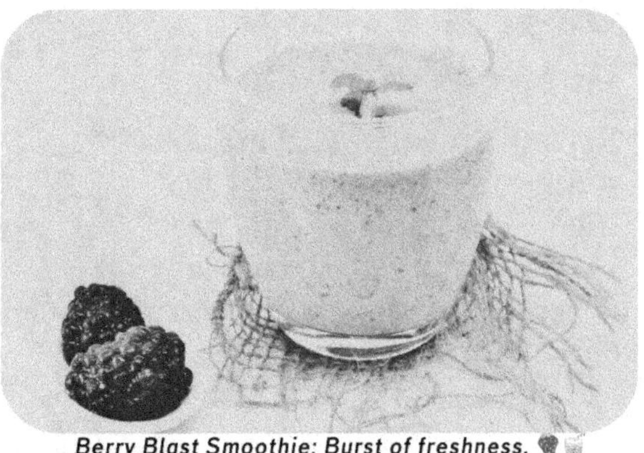

Berry Blast Smoothie: Burst of freshness.

INGREDIENTS:

- 1 cup mixed berries (strawberries, blueberries, raspberries)
- 1/2 frozen banana (for creamier texture).
- 1/2 cup Greek yogurt or dairy-free substitute.
- 1 spoonful of chia seeds
- 1 cup almond milk (or other chosen drink)
- Ice cubes (Optional)

INSTRUCTIONS

1. In a blender, combine mixed berries, bananas, Greek yogurt, chia seeds, and almond milk.
2. Blend until smooth and creamy.
3. If you prefer a colder consistency, add more ice cubes.
4. Pour into a glass and enjoy the blast of fruit flavor.

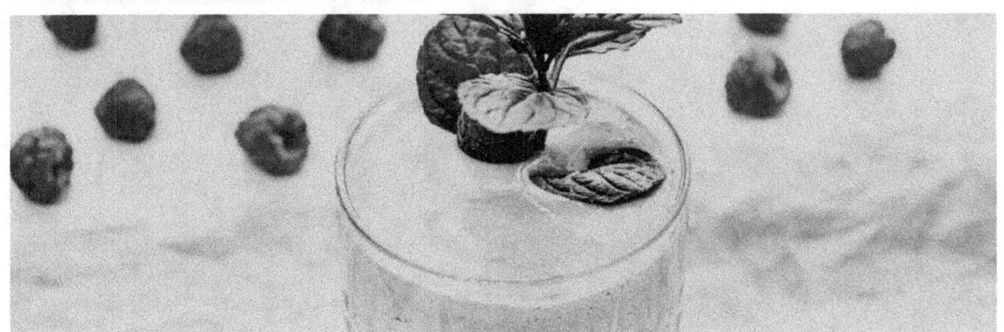

Sip on this delicious Berry Blast Smoothie, which is high in antioxidants and important minerals. Add a handful of almonds for extra protein to make a tasty and PCOS-friendly breakfast or snack.

Prep ⏰
5 minutes

Cook ⏰
0 minutes

Serves
4

Ginger & Lemon Detox Water

Refresh your hydration routine with this PCOS-friendly Ginger Lemon Detox Water. This beverage is packed with zesty flavors and is intended to help you feel better.

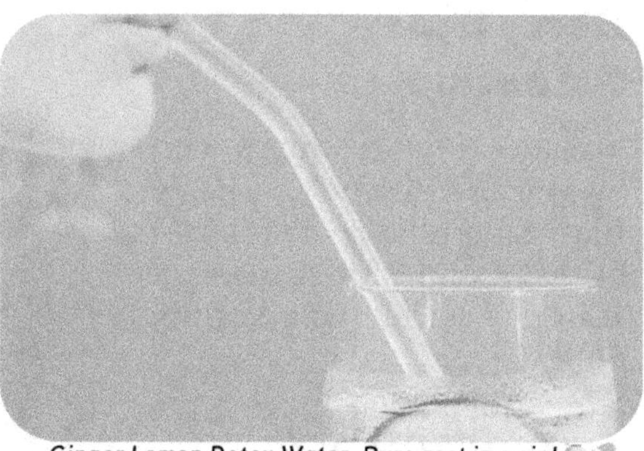

Ginger Lemon Detox Water. Pure zest in a sip!

INGREDIENTS:

- 1 tablespoon freshly grated ginger
- 1 thinly sliced lemon
- Mint leaves (optional)
- 1-2 liters of water

INSTRUCTIONS

1. In a pitcher, combine the freshly grated ginger, lemon slices, and mint leaves.
2. Fill the pitcher with water.
3. Refrigerate for at least 2 hours or overnight to let the ingredients permeate.
4. Serve over ice and savor the crisp, purifying flavor.

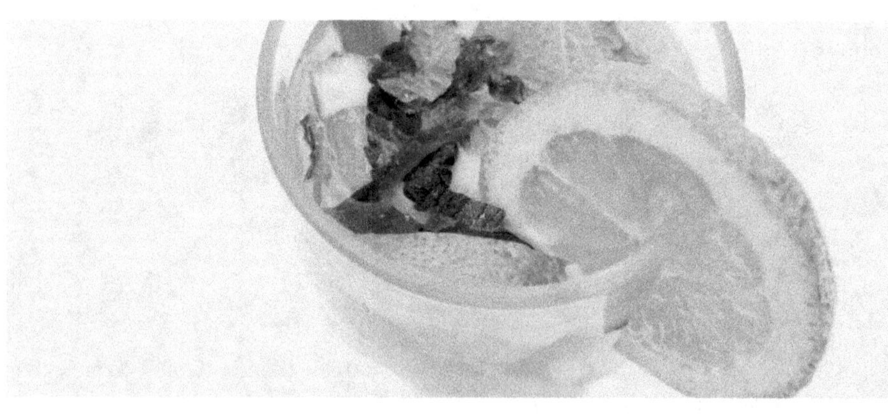

Indulge in the goodness of my Ginger Lemon Detox Water to stay hydrated and energetic. This detox water pairs well with light salads or grilled chicken, making it an excellent choice for a nutritious and PCOS-friendly lunch.

Prep ⏲	**Cook** ⏲	**Serves**
5 minutes	0 minutes	2

Citrus Mint Refresher

Quench your thirst with a rush of freshness! My Citrus Mint Refresher is a refreshing beverage that not only keeps you hydrated but also adds zest to your day. This beverage, packed with citrusy flavor and a dash of mint, is a welcome addition to your PCOS-friendly drink menu.

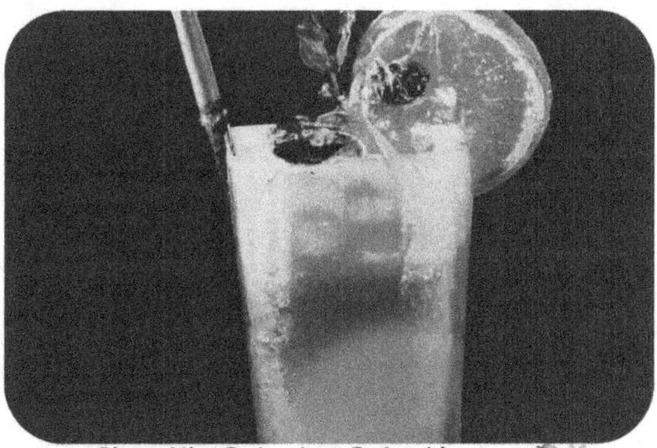

Citrus Mint Refresher: Refreshing zest.

INGREDIENTS:

- 1 juiced orange
- 1 juiced lime
- A handful of fresh mint leaves
- 2 cups cold water
- Ice cubes.
- Honey or other natural sweetener (optional)

INSTRUCTIONS

1. In a pitcher, mix the orange juice, lime juice, and fresh mint leaves.
2. Add cold water and mix thoroughly.
3. Refrigerate for at least 30 minutes to let the flavors to combine.
4. Pour over ice and top with honey if desired.

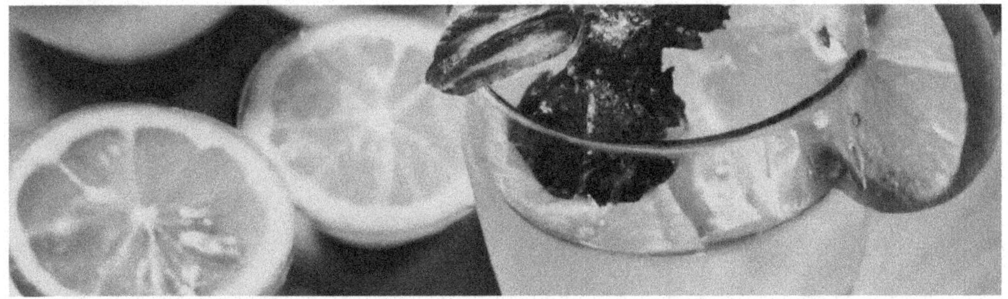

This Citrus Mint Refresher will keep you feeling refreshed and invigorated. This PCOS-friendly drink combines the zesty flavors of orange and lime with the energizing perfume of fresh mint. Whether you're drinking it by the pool or at your desk, this beverage is a delicious way to stay cool and energized. Cheers to a sip-worthy and healthy hydration!

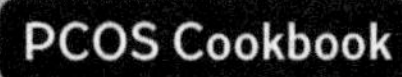

12

Weekly Meal Plans

Embark on a journey of delicious and PCOS-friendly eating with my Weekly Meal Plans. This section caters to diverse preferences, offering balanced meal plans tailored to your taste. Additionally, discover helpful Grocery Shopping Tips to make your journey toward a healthier lifestyle even more seamless. Let's make meal planning an enjoyable and nourishing part of your week!

Balanced Meal Plans for Different Preferences

Embark on a four-week of balanced and PCOS-friendly eating with my carefully crafted meal plans designed to accommodate different preferences. Whether you're a vegetarian, a lover of lean proteins, or prefer plant-based options, these meal plans cater to various tastes while ensuring your nutritional needs are met. Get ready to enjoy a diverse and delightful range of meals that make managing PCOS a delicious part of your lifestyle!

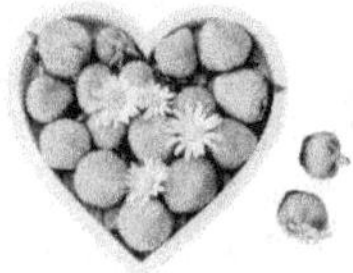

Weekly Meal Plan

Week 1; Varied Vegetarian Delights

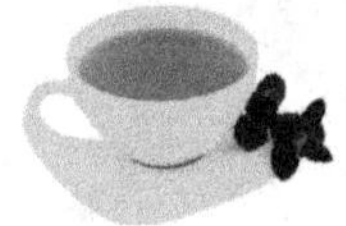

DAY 1

Breakfast	Lunch	Dinner	Snacks
Yogurt Parfait with Berries and Almonds	Chickpea and Spinach Curry	Lentil and Vegetable Soup	Hummus with Veggie Sticks

DAY 2

Breakfast	Lunch	Dinner	Snacks
Chia Seed Pudding with Mixed Fruit	Spinach and Feta Stuffed Portobello Mushrooms	Zucchini Noodles with Pesto	Almond and Coconut Energy Bites

DAY 3

Breakfast	Lunch	Dinner	Snacks
Green Tea Infusion & Whole Grain Toast with Avocado	Quinoa Salad with Roasted Veggies	Cauliflower & Chickpea Curry	Greek Yogurt & Berry Parfait

DAY 4

Breakfast	Lunch	Dinner	Snacks
Quinoa Power Bowl with Fresh Fruits	Sweet Potato & Chickpea Patties	Tomato Avocado Bruschetta	Spicy Roasted Chickpeas

DAY 5

Breakfast	Lunch	Dinner	Snacks
Berry Blast Smoothie Bowl	Quinoa & Black Bean Pilaf	Grilled Portobello Mushrooms with Garlic & Herbs	Popcorn with Turmeric and Paprika

DAY 6

Breakfast	Lunch	Dinner	Snacks
Avocado & Berry Smoothie Bowl	Chickpea & Spinach Salad	Eggplant Lasagna	Balsamic Glazed Carrots

DAY 7

Breakfast	Lunch	Dinner	Snacks
Overnight Oats with Mixed Berries	Kale & Cranberry Salad	Quinoa & Roasted Vegetable Buddha Bowl	Lemon Herb Asparagus

Weekly Meal Plan

Week 2: Protein-Packed Pleasures

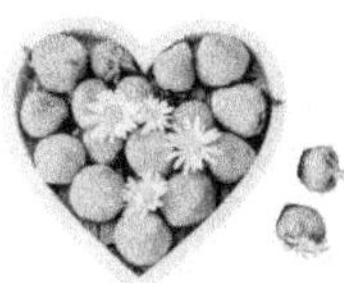
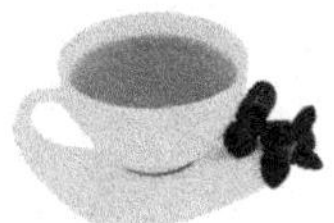

DAY 1

Breakfast	Lunch	Dinner	Snacks
Berry Blast Smoothie	Turkey & Quinoa Stuffed Peppers	Tofu Stir-Fry with Broccoli	Edamame Hummus with Veggie Sticks

DAY 2

Breakfast	Lunch	Dinner	Snacks
Scrambled Eggs with Spinach & Tomatoes	Quinoa Power Salad	Baked Chicken with Roasted Vegetables	Almond Butter Banana Bites

DAY 3

Breakfast	Lunch	Dinner	Snacks
Smoothie Bowl with Mixed Berries & Granola	Lentil & Vegetable Soup	Grilled Salmon with Quinoa Pilaf	Popcorn with Turmeric & Paprika

DAY 4

Breakfast	Lunch	Dinner	Snacks
Greek Yogurt Parfait with Mixed Berries	Tomato Basil Zoodle Soup	Spinach & Feta Stuffed Mushrooms	Almond & Coconut Energy Bites

DAY 5

Breakfast	Lunch	Dinner	Snacks
Chia Seed Pudding with Berries	Chickpea & Spinach Curry	Lemon Herb Baked Chicken	Garlic Roasted Brussels Sprouts

DAY 6

Breakfast	Lunch	Dinner	Snacks
Avocado & Berry Smoothie Bowl	Quinoa & Black Bean Pilaf	Grilled Portobello Mushrooms with Garlic & Herbs	Mashed Sweet Potatoes

DAY 7

Breakfast	Lunch	Dinner	Snacks
Overnight Oats with Mixed Berries	Kale & Cranberry Salad	Quinoa & Roasted Vegetable Buddha Bowl	Lemon Herb Asparagus

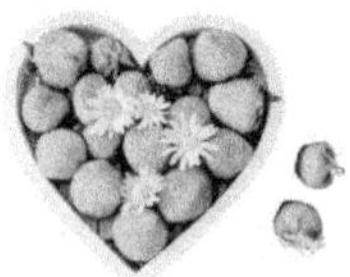
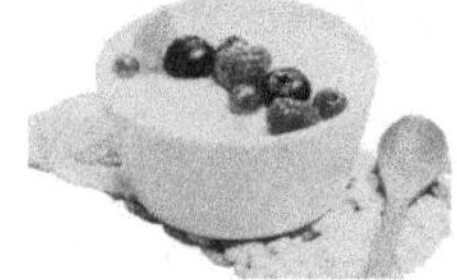

Weekly Meal Plan

Week 3: Plant-Powered Bliss

DAY 1

Breakfast	Lunch	Dinner	Snacks
Avocado & Berry Smoothie Bowl	Sweet Potato & Chickpea Patties	Cauliflower & Chickpea Curry	Spicy Roasted Chickpeas

DAY 2

Breakfast	Lunch	Dinner	Snacks
Citrus Shrimp Salad	Eggplant Lasagna	Chickpea & Spinach Curry	Quinoa & Black Bean Pilaf

DAY 3

Breakfast	Lunch	Dinner	Snacks
Kale & Cranberry Salad	Balsamic Glazed Carrots	Quinoa Salad with Roasted Veggies	Almond & Coconut Energy Bites

DAY 4

Breakfast	Lunch	Dinner	Snacks
Chia Seed Pudding with Berries	Lentil & Vegetable Soup	Grilled Salmon with Lemon Dill Sauce	Popcorn with Turmeric & Paprika

DAY 5

Breakfast	Lunch	Dinner	Snacks
Greek Yogurt Parfait with Mixed Berries	Lemon Herb Asparagus	Spinach & Feta Stuffed Portobello Mushrooms	Almond Butter Banana Bites

DAY 6

Breakfast	Lunch	Dinner	Snacks
Quinoa Power Salad	Mashed Sweet Potatoes	Dark Chocolate Avocado Mousse	Garlic Roasted Brussels Sprouts

DAY 7

Breakfast	Lunch	Dinner	Snacks
Coconut & Berry Parfait	Quinoa & Roasted Vegetable Buddha Bowl	Zucchini Noodles with Pesto	Snack: Edamame Hummus with Veggie Sticks

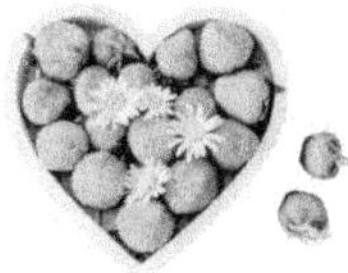
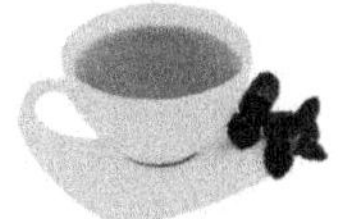

Weekly Meal Plan

Week 4: Flavorful Plant-Based Delights

DAY 1

Breakfast	Lunch	Dinner	Snacks
Avocado Toast with Cherry Tomatoes	Lentil and Vegetable Stew	Sweet Potato & Chickpea Curry	Fresh Fruit Salad

DAY 2

Breakfast	Lunch	Dinner	Snacks
Green Smoothie with Spinach, Banana, & Almond Milk	Quinoa Salad with Roasted Veggies	Zucchini Noodles with Tomato Basil Sauce	Hummus with Sliced Cucumber

DAY 3

Breakfast	Lunch	Dinner	Snacks
Chia Seed Pudding with Mango	Spinach & Feta Stuffed Portobello Mushrooms	Chickpea and Spinach Curry	Almond & Coconut Energy Bites

DAY 4

Breakfast	Lunch	Dinner	Snacks
Smoothie Bowl with Mixed Berries & Granola	Kale and Cranberry Salad	Eggplant Lasagna	Greek Yogurt and Berry Parfait

DAY 5

Breakfast	Lunch	Dinner	Snacks
Whole Grain Toast with Peanut Butter & Banana	Quinoa Power Salad	Cauliflower and Chickpea Stir-Fry	Spicy Roasted Chickpeas

DAY 6

Breakfast	Lunch	Dinner	Snacks
Berry Smoothie Bowl	Tomato Basil Zoodle Soup	Quinoa Stuffed Bell Peppers	Mixed Nuts and Seeds

DAY 7

Breakfast	Lunch	Dinner	Snacks
Overnight Oats with Chia Seeds & Berries	Roasted Beet & Goat Cheese Salad	Lentil & Vegetable Stir-Fry	Sliced Apple with Almond Butter

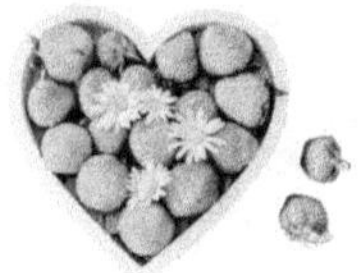

Weekly Meal Plan

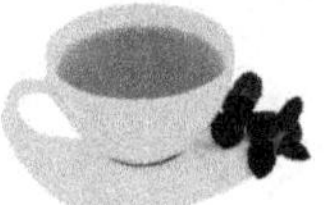

Note: The meal plan is a starting point, and you're encouraged to mix and match recipes based on your preferences. Remember to stay hydrated and listen to your body. Your well-being is at the heart of these culinary creations. Cheers to a healthier and delicious lifestyle! Happy cooking!

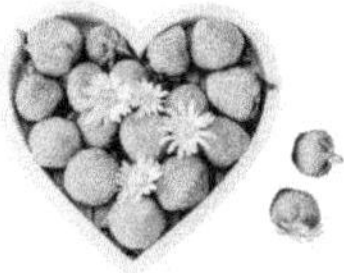

Weekly Meal Plan

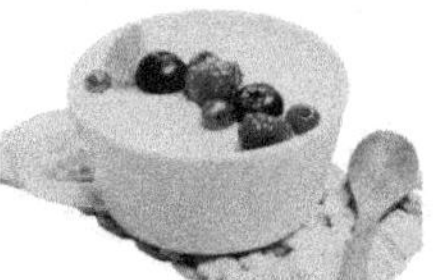

Week:

D A Y 1

Breakfast	Lunch	Dinner	Snacks

D A Y 2

Breakfast	Lunch	Dinner	Snacks

D A Y 3

Breakfast	Lunch	Dinner	Snacks

D A Y 4

Breakfast	Lunch	Dinner	Snacks

D A Y 5

Breakfast	Lunch	Dinner	Snacks

D A Y 6

Breakfast	Lunch	Dinner	Snacks

D A Y 7

Breakfast	Lunch	Dinner	Snacks

PCOS Grocery Shopping Tips 

Grocery shopping for PCOS can be both efficient and beneficial. Here are some detailed purchasing tips:

- **Whole Foods**. First, focus on complete, pure meals. Fresh fruits and vegetables, lean proteins, and nutritious grains should make up the majority of your shopping cart.
- **Colorful Produce**: Choose a variety of colorful fruits and vegetables. These contain antioxidants, vitamins, and minerals that can benefit overall health.
- **Select lean proteins**. Include lean protein sources such as chicken, fish, tofu, and lentils. They give essential nutrients while limiting saturated fat.
- **I like complex carbs**: Choose whole grains instead of processed carbs. Quinoa, brown rice, and oats are high-fiber foods that provide continuous energy.
- **Healthful Fats**: Consume healthy fats such as avocados, nuts, seeds, and olive oil. These can assist to keep hormones in balance.
- **Mindful Dairy Choices**: Choose dairy or low-fat options. Some PCOS sufferers may choose lactose-free or plant-based alternatives.
- **Reduce processed foods**. Cut back on processed and sugary foods. These can induce insulin resistance, which is a serious concern among PCOS patients.
- **Check the labels**: Check labels for hidden sugars, spurious substances, and bad fats. Look for items with fewer components.
- **Coffee and Hydration**: Enjoy coffee in moderation and drink plenty of water. Herbal teas are also a great option.

- **Plan and List**: Prepare a weekly menu and grocery list. This allows you to stay on track, minimize impulse purchases, and make sure you have all of the components for your PCOS-friendly recipes.
- **Eat Balanced Meals**: Make sure your meals are rich in protein, healthy fats, and complex carbohydrates. This promotes regular blood sugar levels.
- **Mindful Snacking**: Choose nutritious snacks such as fresh fruits, vegetables with hummus, or a handful of nuts. Be cautious with serving sizes.
- **Frozen fruit and vegetables**:
- Fruit and vegetables can be frozen. They are more convenient, have a longer shelf life, and are equally healthy as fresh ones.
- **Cost-effective Options**: Healthy eating doesn't have to be expensive. Look for sales, buy in quantity, and consider seasonal produce to get the greatest deal.
- **Ask a Nutritionist**: Speak with a nutritionist or healthcare professional to get specialized recommendations tailored to your specific needs and preferences.

With these strategies, grocery shopping will become a proactive step toward better PCOS health. Have fun shopping! 🛒🍎

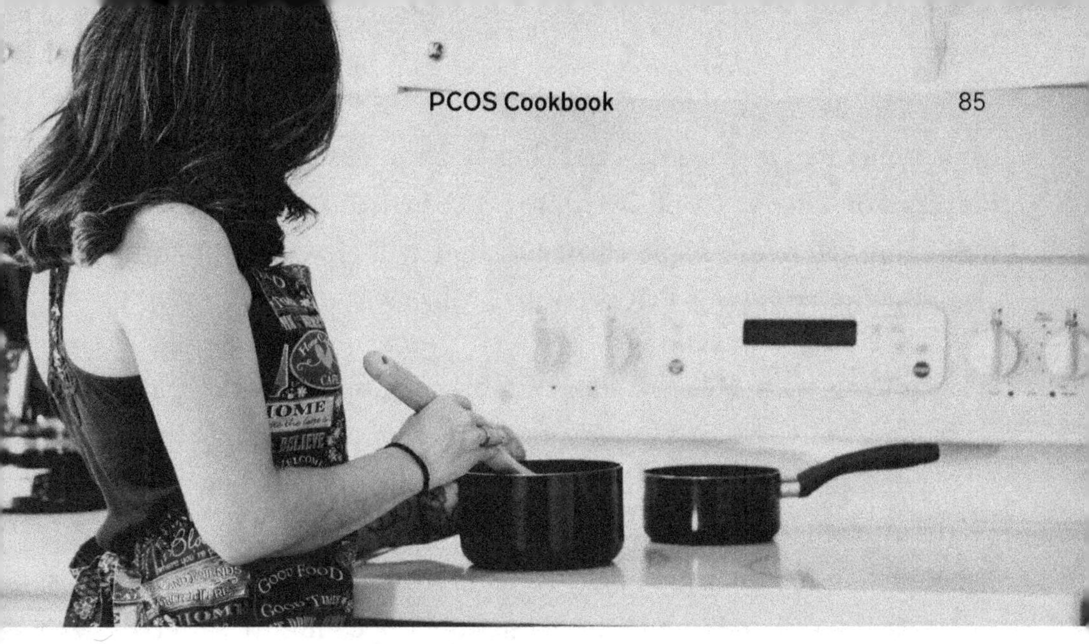

13

Kitchen Tricks: My PCOS-Friendly Culinary Haven

Embarking on a PCOS-friendly culinary adventure is more than simply recipes; it's a comprehensive strategy that begins in the heart of your home: the kitchen. In this part, I'm pleased to provide some kitchen tips for PCOS fighters.

Join me as we unearth the secrets of PCOS-friendly cooking, changing your kitchen into a place where flavor, health, and empowerment coexist harmoniously.

PCOS-Friendly Cooking Techniques:

Learn about cooking techniques that use PCOS-friendly ingredients. From sautéing to roasting, these methods not only improve flavor but also keep the nutritious value your body need.

Mastering PCOS-friendly cooking techniques is like opening a universe of culinary options that are beneficial to your health and well-being. Here are some strategies that will elevate your food while also aligning with your PCOS control journey:

1. **Sautéing with Healthy Fats**: Embrace sautéing with healthy fats such as olive oil or avocado oil. This approach retains the aromas of the ingredients while supplying necessary nutrients for PCOS treatment.

2. **Roasting for Intense Flavor**: Roasting veggies or proteins enhances their flavors, making them irresistibly appealing. It's a terrific way to improve the taste without sacrificing nutrition.

3. **Steaming for nutrient retention**: Steaming might help you retain nutrients. This gentle cooking approach preserves your vegetables' nutritional value, providing a health boost with each bite.

4. **Grilling for Lean Options**: Grilling is ideal for preparing lean, flavorful meals. This technique gives a smokey flavor to veggies or lean protein sources such as chicken or fish without using too much fat.

5. **Baking With Wholesome Ingredients**: Choose baking as a way to make PCOS-friendly goodies. To keep your baked goods nutritious, use whole grain flours, natural sugars, and nutrient-dense ingredients.

By combining these cooking techniques into your culinary arsenal, you are not only preparing meals, but also creating foods that will help your PCOS journey. Enjoy cooking while nourishing your body.

Essential pantry items

Stocking your cupboard with the necessary ingredients might make or break your PCOS-friendly cooking experience. Discover a carefully curated selection of must-have ingredients that serve as the foundation for delicious and healthy meals. Let me transform your kitchen into a PCOS-friendly utopia, one pantry item at a time.

Join me as we unearth the secrets of PCOS-friendly cooking, changing your kitchen into a place where flavor, health, and empowerment coexist harmoniously.

Building a PCOS-friendly pantry is an important step toward achieving your health and wellbeing objectives. Here's a comprehensive list of pantry staples that are PCOS-friendly:

Whole Grains:

- Brown Rice: A healthy alternative to white rice, high in fiber and minerals.
- Quinoa: A complete protein source with a low glycemic index, which aids in blood sugar regulation.
- Oats: High in soluble fiber, which aids digestion and provides a consistent source of energy.

Healthy Fats:

- Olive Oil: Rich in monounsaturated fats, which promote heart health.
- Avocado Oil: High in oleic acid, which promotes cardiovascular health and reduces inflammation.
- Nuts and Seeds: Almonds, walnuts, chia seeds, and flaxseeds are rich in healthful fats, fiber, and omega-3 fatty acids.

Lean Protein:

- Lean Poultry: Skinless chicken and turkey breast are high-protein selections.
- Fatty Fish: Salmon and mackerel contain omega-3 fatty acids, which promote heart health.
- Plant-Based Proteins: Use legumes, lentils, and chickpeas as vegetarian protein sources.

Low glycemic sweeteners:

- Stevia: A natural sweetener with no calories and minimal effect on blood sugar.
- Honey: A natural sweetener that contains antioxidants and may have anti-inflammatory properties.

Herbs and Spices:

- Turmeric: Well-known for its anti-inflammatory qualities.
- Cinnamon: May help control blood sugar levels.
- Ginger: Improves digestion and contains anti-inflammatory properties.

Canned & Dried Goods:

- Canned Tomatoes: A diverse base for sauces and high in antioxidants like lycopene.
- Legumes: Include canned chickpeas, black beans, and lentils for easy protein options.

Whole Grain Flours:

- Whole Wheat Flour: A fiber-rich option for baking.
- Almond Flour: This gluten-free choice has a nutty flavor.

Non-Dairy Alternatives

- Almond Milk or Coconut Milk: Low in calories and a good substitute for dairy.

Whole fruits & vegetables

- Fresh or frozen: Make sure you have a choice of colorful foods high in vitamins and minerals.

Teas & Infusions

- Green Tea: Packed with antioxidants and perhaps advantageous to metabolic health.

Dark Chocolate:

- 70% Cocoa or More: A moderate amount can deliver antioxidants while requiring less sugar.

Creating a well-stocked pantry with these necessities ensures that you have a solid basis for making various and nutritious PCOS meals. To maintain a healthy diet, inspect and replace your pantry on a regular basis.

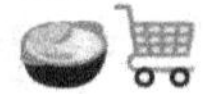

Prep ⏰
5 minutes

Bunus Recipe

Serves
1

PCOS Power Smoothie Bowl

Embark on a tasty adventure with my extra recipe, the PCOS Power Smoothie Bowl! This bright dish is more than just a tasty treat; it's also a nutritious powerhouse meant to compliment your PCOS-friendly lifestyle. It's packed with kale, berries, chia seeds, and a hint of almond butter, making it the ideal way to start your day with a boost of energy and health.

INGREDIENTS:

- 1 cup kale leaves (stems removed)
- 1/2 cup mixed berries (strawberries, blueberries, raspberries)
- 1 tablespoon chia seeds.
- 1/2 frozen banana.
- 1 tablespoon of almond butter. 1/2 cup unsweetened almond milk
- Choose your own toppings: Sliced strawberries, chia seeds, and granola

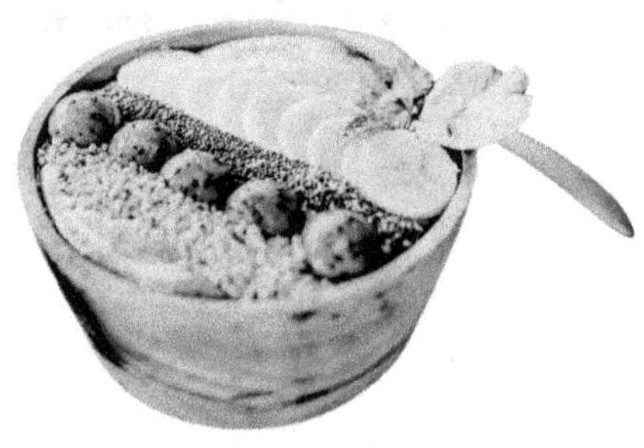

INSTRUCTIONS

1. Blend together kale, mixed berries, chia seeds, frozen banana, almond butter, and almond milk.
2. Blend until smooth and creamy, adding more almond milk as needed.
3. Pour the smoothie into a bowl and top with your favorite toppings, such as sliced strawberries, chia seeds, and granola.
4. Use a spoon to relish the nutrient-packed bliss!

As you enjoy this PCOS Power Smoothie Bowl, keep in mind that you are not only indulging your taste buds, but also fueling your health. Feel free to add extra toppings like shredded coconut or a spray of honey. It's a treat for you, a delicious way to commemorate your path to wellness. Enjoy! 🌿

DEDICATION

To every journey toward wellness and the strength that comes from loving and caring for our bodies. This cookbook is devoted to everyone on the path to PCOS wellness. May these dishes add joy, flavor, and a sense of empowerment to your culinary excursions. Best wishes for your unique and wonderful journey! 🌿🥥.

Delve Deeper

Check out this link: https://www.amazon.com/author/dixon-d or scan the QR Code below to delve deeper
into the world of wellness with my companion book, Low Carb Diet, which is a vital element of the 'Savor & Thrive' series. Discover a variety of low-carb culinary delights to complement your path to health and vigor.

Whether you're a seasoned health enthusiast or just starting out on your wellness journey, this book provides practical ideas, delectable recipes, and a road map to enjoying the benefits of a low-carb lifestyle. Together with the rest of the 'Savor & Thrive' series, it invites you to relish each meal while also thriving on your wellness journey.

Improve your health, one tasty meal at a time. Discover the benefits of low-carb living through the rich tapestry of the 'Savor & Thrive' series, where each recipe is a step toward a more vibrant you.